The Foundations of Emergency Care

The Foundations of Emergency Care

Edited by Cliff Evans and Emma Tippins

Open University Press

Open University Press
McGraw-Hill Education
McGraw-Hill House
Shoppenhangers Road
Maidenhead
Berkshire
England
SL6 2QL

email: enquiries@openup.co.uk
world wide web: www.openup.co.uk

and Two Penn Plaza, New York, NY 10121-2289, USA

First published 2007

A catalogue record of this book is available from the British Library

ISBN-10: 0 335 22124 6 (pb)   0 335 22125 4 (hb)
ISBN-13: 978 0 335 221240 (pb)   978 0 335 22125 7 (hb)

Library of Congress Cataloging-in-Publication Data
CIP data applied for

Typeset by RefineCatch Limited, Bungay, Suffolk
Printed by Bell & Bain Ltd, Glasgow

The *McGraw·Hill* Companies

Contents

List of contributors

Cliff Evans is an Emergency Care Lecturer at Thames Valley University, facilitating pre-registration nurses in critical care skills and post-registration nurses into gaining advanced clinical knowledge and skills towards specialist degrees in both emergency care and acute cardiology.

Andrew Frazer is a Consultant Nurse at the Accident and Emergency Department, Newham University Hospital Trust, and Honorary Lecturer at City University. Andrew is also an ATNC/ALS instructor and manages a clinical caseload of major's patients, and has responsibilities for both education and research.

Jayne Gwyther is a Practice Facilitator within Bro Morgannwg NHS Trust, providing academic teaching and support for mentors and students within the clinical area. Jayne also teaches across both adult and child branches of the curriculum and has a specific interest in child health teaching and recognition of the critically ill child.

Paul Newcombe is a Senior Lecturer at Kingston University and St George's, University of London, and delivers core emergency care education to emergency nurses in south-west London.

Michelle Stanton is a Clinical Nurse Specialist in Family Planning Nursing. She will be completing her MEd (ICT) in July 2006. Michelle is Programme Leader for the Breast and Cervical Cancer Screening Course and Senior Lecturer in Adult Health Nursing at Thames Valley University, London. Her job also involves e-learning design, development and online tutoring.

Emma Tippins is a modern matron, fulfilling both clinical and managerial roles at Heatherwood and Wexham Park Hospitals NHS Trust. Emma is also an advanced life support and advanced trauma nursing course instructor and has an MSc in Advancing Critical Care Practice.

Claire Washbourne specializes in emergency medicine and has worked in hospitals in London and Australia. Claire currently works as a Consultant Nurse for Minor Injury & Illness in the Emergency Department at Chelsea & Westminster Hospital NHS Trust. Part of her role includes teaching and the clinical support of nursing and medical staff, as well as treating patients autonomously, including independent nurse prescribing within the Emergency Nurse Practitioner service.

Foreword

Emma Tippins and I have specialized in both acute and emergency care for several years. Emma is currently in the role of Matron for Emergency Care, a role that encompasses the local application of national strategies aimed at ensuring the provision of the highest standards of patient care. I work as an emergency care lecturer, which includes teaching pre-registration nurses critical care skills and facilitating post-registration nurses working in the speciality of emergency care in becoming emergency care specialists. In my opinion, there is a distinct difference between the two: specialists are dynamic, and able to take the initiative when faced with clinical dilemmas. Their clinical decision-making and practice are amenable to questioning and change, specialists seek ways to improve the experience of those they care for by adapting to suit their current circumstance. This centres on the ability of the practitioner to take ownership of their own professional development and seek ways of increasing their knowledge base, thereby providing patients with an improved level of care. This is not an overnight accomplishment; in fact, despite a solid foundation of theoretical understanding the application of this knowledge into clinical practice can take years.

Emergency care, wherever the location, offers practitioners the chance to play a pivotal role in the care of their local community, and the importance of these primary interventions cannot be over-emphasized, as many emergency presentations would not reach secondary care without them.

We wanted to write a book that offered the reader a unique insight into how experienced emergency care providers approach patient care, demonstrating how they establish their plan of treatment: not on subjective opinion, but on objective data and evidence-based protocols.

My initial concept was to produce a book that students, inexperienced practitioners or those wanting to apply an evidence base to their practice could utilize while at work, to assist with problem-solving and provide easily identified rationales to common patient presentations. Later the reader could reflect on their clinical encounters and gain further insight into the relevant pathophysiology, statistics and treatment options.

There are of course thousands of potential presentations and in order for the book to be a portable companion, these had to be limited. The identified areas of practice pinpoint either common patient presentations, where the practitioner can have a particularly powerful influence on the patient outcome, or those presentations where the management protocols are based on quantifiable evidence.

In our opinion, the areas highlighted within this book will guide those new to emergency care, or those wanting to improve their assessment skills, towards gaining a solid foundation of theoretical knowledge and clinical guidance on common clinical conditions that will ultimately improve the patient experience.

The following chapters are written by an incredible array of practitioners including consultant nurses, lecturers and modern matrons, all of whom directly influence modern strategy and practice. It is therefore our pleasure to introduce this book to the reader and to thank the contributors for providing an excellent insight into their everyday practice.

Cliff Evans

Acknowledgements

We would like to thank Christopher Robinson and Ian O'Reilly at TVU Media for their help and ideas on illustrations used within this book, and Georgina White for her technical assistance. A special thank you goes to Andrew Frazer for stepping into this project at a late stage, and to Rachel Crookes for her support and encouragement, without whom this project would never have materialized.

Cliff Evans and Emma Tippins

1   Introduction to emergency care

Emma Tippins and Cliff Evans

Emergency care

Emergency Care is politically and socially one of the highest priorities in society today. Increasing patient expectations and the advancement in scientific and medical knowledge have had a dramatic effect on the provision of emergency care. The Department of Health's (DoH) White Paper on Reforming Emergency Care (2001) stipulates that emergency care provision should address the demands and needs of patients, regardless of setting. A solid foundational knowledge in the skills of triage and assessment are, therefore, essential precursors to all emergency practitioners in order to enable patients to be treated quickly, appropriately and effectively, i.e., right skill, right time, right place. The different, diverse and unique needs of patients provide a constant challenge to emergency practitioners.

The Emergency Department (ED) is the portal for over 16.5 million annual visits in England (Alberti 2004). In the United States of America (USA) there are over 100 million annual visits, accounting for 40 per cent of hospital admissions (McCaig and Burt 1999). These millions of patients will attend with any number of clinical presentations and complaints requiring the assistance of every medical speciality. The role of the emergency practitioner is unique in this respect, as in no other clinical setting will clinicians be called upon to assess and identify the needs of such a wide range of potential patient conditions.

The ED is commonly the interface between patients and emergency care, within this setting a patient's first contact with a healthcare professional will usually be at the point of initial assessment; the process of triage. Triage is a dynamic decision-making process that will prioritize an individual's need for treatment on their presenting history, the nature of the incident, and the presenting clinical complaint. An efficient triage system aims to identify and expedite time-critical treatment for patients with life-threatening conditions, and ensure every patient requiring emergency treatment is prioritized according to their clinical need. The ethos of triage systems relates to the ability of a professional to detect critical illness, which has to be balanced with resource implications of 'over-triage' (a triage category of higher acuity is allocated). A decision that underestimates a person's level of clinical urgency may delay time-critical interventions; furthermore, prolonged triage processes may contribute to adverse patient outcomes (Geraci and Geraci 1994; Travers 1999), and impede the assessment of others.

In this context, the practitioner's ability to take an accurate patient history, conduct a brief physical assessment, and rapidly determine clinical urgency are crucial to the provision of safe and efficient emergency care (Travers 1999). These responsibilities require practitioners undertaking triage to justify their clinical decisions with evidence from clinical research, and to be accountable for decisions they make within the clinical environment.

This book is directed at facilitating front-line practitioners and students aiming to specialize within emergency care, to gain the essential assessment skills necessary for acute care environments, and to forge a solid foundation of theoretical knowledge and understanding upon which to base their clinical practice.

Applying theory to practice

In order to deliver expert individualized care, emergency care providers need to make multiple decisions rapidly, in highly complex environments and under increasing pressure. Emergency care is a dynamic specialism very different from many other areas of care provision, yet the skills associated with emergency care can be applied to all acute areas. Patients often present critically ill and frequently highly unstable, as a result, their rapidly changing conditions demand intelligent and decisive decision-making from practitioners in short time frames. Despite this, there remains minimal research on the clinical decision-making skills of emergency care providers. Consequently much of the content and structure of the decision-making process remains unclear (Fonteyn and Ritter 2000).

Clinical decision-making can be defined as the process practitioners use to gather patient information, evaluate that information and make a judgement that results in the provision of patient care (Andersson et al. 2006). This process involves collecting information through the use of both scientific and intuitive assessment skills. This information is then interpreted through the use of knowledge and past experiences (Cioffi 2000; Tippins 2005).

Recent research indicates that many practitioners have a solid foundation of theoretical knowledge but often fail to apply this knowledge directly to patient care (Tippins 2005). The Resuscitation Council, European and UK, have acknowledged this phenomenon based on several research studies identifying that up to two-thirds of in-hospital cardiac arrests are potentially avoidable (Franklin and Matthew 1994; Hodgetts et al. 2002). Seeking to address these issues, the DoH set national guidelines, stating that all healthcare providers should receive competency-based high dependency training (DoH 2000). Universities introduced higher educational modules attempting to facilitate experienced and novice post-registration practitioners into gaining these fundamental skills associated with the process of initial and ongoing patient assessment. This essential ability to recognize both patients at risk of critical illness and sudden physical deterioration, and those actually experiencing critical illness is now an indispensable component of modules which all pre-registration nurses have to pass in order to register in the UK (NMC 2004).

The recently revised Resuscitation Guidelines (RCUK) 2006) directly address the DoH's objectives by focusing on the recognition and treatment of the critically ill patient in order to prevent cardiac arrest. This focus on preventative education has seen the development of locally delivered courses such as the Acute Life Threatening Events: Recognition and Treatment (ALERT) course, and the development of early warning scores (EWS). Within the UK EWS are now commonly used to identify patients at risk of clinical deterioration. The use of an EWS ensures a structured approach to patient assessment and the regular recording of physiological observations, a crucial first step in recognizing patients at risk. Physical parameters are used to identify patients who are deteriorating, or are at risk of doing so. The scoring system alerts the carer to the potential for serious illness and initiates a call for senior assistance.

Regardless of the individual setting, practitioners encountering acutely ill patients need to be able to identify those at risk of serious illness, act on these findings and evaluate their chosen treatment route. Although these key skills may be used in other clinical settings, they are essential to emergency care provision and are seen as an integral part of an acute practitioner's scope of clinical practice.

Emergency care management is a complex and dynamic specialism. The role of the emergency practitioner comprises numerous fundamental clinical skills. Practitioners, regardless of their discipline, need the ability to relate these skills, including a foundational knowledge of the physical changes synonymous with serious illness, to the patient assessment process. This can be achieved by applying the key skills of critical thinking and analysis to everyday clinical decision-making.

The argument surrounding the clinical application of theoretical knowledge has continued throughout nursing and healthcare education. The NHS Plan (DoH 2000) identified the NHS as deficient in national evidence-based standards and, therefore, much of the practice subjective to individual interpretation. This initiated the current protocol-driven approach to care which aims to provide practitioners, and subsequently patients, with evidence-based objective treatment regimens, in contrast to individual subjective preferences. A prime example is demonstrated by the advanced life support algorithms, which have revolutionized multi-disciplinary care delivery.

Changing practice within the vast institution of healthcare is a monumental task and to this end clinical governance was established. The clinical governance initiative is conveyed into clinical practice by the National Institute of Health and Clinical Excellence (NICE). NICE, in conjunction with several specialist professional institutions, have released numerous national guidelines on specific patient presentations or illnesses. These are also supplemented by the DoH's National Service Frameworks (NSF), which set clinical standards in relation to specific disorders and specialist organizations such as the British Thoracic Society, which promote 'best-practice'. These initiatives have combined to produce a constantly progressive clinical arena in which novice practitioners and students can easily become lost.

There is, therefore, a clear need to apply a tool or structure to the diagnostic process directly aimed at facilitating practitioners with the ability to base their clinical findings on objective rather than subjective data. This facilitation centres on two components: first, a solid understanding of the signs and symptoms associated with physical illness, and second, the application of critical thinking to their practice. The first component is demonstrated throughout this book by experienced practitioners who discuss their own experiences in the form of patient scenarios which highlight both common clinical encounters and the frameworks and protocols they use to prioritize, and manage, patients quickly, appropriately and effectively. In addition, the clinicians discuss the associated anatomy and physiology providing the reader with several key words or triggers. This enquiry-based learning approach promotes lifelong learning by encouraging the reader to seek key texts listed at the end of each chapter, thereby gaining further knowledge and understanding of the topics.

The framework used throughout this book is based on a modification of Alfaro-LeFevre's (2004) approach to critical thinking, the DEAD framework. Novice practitioners frequently require an unambiguous approach to patient assessment, which can be achieved by applying the DEAD acronym. This framework not only aids practitioners in critically analysing their care delivery, it also directly provides a safety net by leading the practitioner to question other possibilities regarding the patient presentation, and this component is paramount to those working in acute care settings as a missed diagnosis can be fatal. This structured approach is applied to everyday clinical presentations via the use of clinical scenarios. The scenarios demonstrate classic emergency care presentations and focus on the practitioner applying their theoretical understanding of both anatomy and physiology to determine an individual's clinical status. The practitioner's assessment plan broadens to encompass a holistic approach by adopting the critical thinking approach that guides the practitioner through four categories, which results in a safe and effective method of identifying critical illness through an elimination of serious pathology. The practitioner will increase their understanding of relevant emergency skills and knowledge by directly seeing the application of theoretical knowledge within clinical practice. The enhancing critical thinking approach encourages the reader to seek further understanding of relevant theory, this follows the Nursing and Midwifery Council guidelines on lifelong learning and the ability of the practitioner to be fit for practice (NMC 2004).

This approach is outlined in Box 1.1.

Box 1.1   The DEAD mnemonic outlined

D   *Data* (scientific facts) – these should be based on the facts the practitioner holds and any other data that can be collected to validate or negate them.

E   *Emotions* (intuition or gut feelings/reactions) – what are your instincts telling you?; how can you consolidate or negate these?

A   *Advantages* – advantages to others that would result from actions the clinician takes, i.e., would an action instigated at the initial assessment improve the patient's prognosis, an example being the dispensing of an anti-platelet drug to a patient experiencing an acute coronary syndrome? The practitioner should also consider that a test requested when the patient presents might hasten their visit and result in an increasingly efficient service.

D   *Disadvantages* (differential diagnoses) – what could go wrong, in the worst case scenario what could this be?; how I can rule this out?

By utilizing this structured framework, those less experienced in critical thinking will have a clear systematic outline to assist them in the organization of their thought processes and subsequent clinical practice. This, in turn, could facilitate the individual development of critical thinking and decision-making-skills.

The focal point of this book is to facilitate practitioners to acquire the essential skills of patient assessment and priority assignment, as these comprehensive skills have been highlighted as being paramount to emergency care providers (DoH 2005).

2 The initial assessment: prioritizing care delivery

Cliff Evans

Introduction

One of the principal skills required by all practitioners working within emergency care is the ability to carry out a timely, but comprehensive patient assessment. The focal point is to ascertain the individual care needs of a patient, and assign a correct level of prioritization to the instigation of a treatment regimen. To function effectively the practitioner requires excellent communication skills, and a thorough understanding of how pathology and trauma can affect the internal environment and its equilibrium (homeostasis) leading to the clinically recognized state of physiological shock.

This chapter, therefore, discusses the assessment process, centring on the identification of the life-threatening presentation of physiological shock. This will be achieved in two stages: first, through analysing the clinical patient assessment process, thereby identifying the prime indicators of serious illness that experienced clinicians look for as part of their initial assessment or triage. These include the history of the presenting problem, or mechanism of injury, and the clinical signs and symptoms, which enable a working diagnosis and several variables to be established (differential diagnoses). Second, several diagnostic investigations are undertaken to either consolidate or negate the evolving working diagnosis (data collection).

Once the clinician has a solid foundational knowledge of how pathology or trauma affect homeostasis, the process of recognizing serious illness becomes straightforward with the identification of the sometimes subtle clinical clues leading to the instigation of the correct prioritization of patient care, and ultimately an improved patient prognosis.

The clinician will gain insight into how physiological shock manifests within the external and internal environment and the relationship this has with physiological vital signs and other clinical assessment characteristics. The combination of gaining these skills, and understanding the differing stages and classifications of physiological shock, while incorporating the enhancing critical thinking framework, will enable the inexperienced practitioner to be able to explore clinical scenarios and work at their own pace towards a higher level of clinical practice and theoretical understanding. When confronted by patients with serious pathologies, the clinician applying critical thinking to their practice will be able to assess, formulate a working diagnosis and instigate appropriate tests in conjunction with a safe and adaptable plan of care. This plan of care is built on scientific fact and the clinician's solid physiological knowledge base through the consolidation/negation process; it is therefore dynamic, and open to further construction/deconstruction or challenge.

Homeostasis

Homeostasis refers to the state of functional equilibrium within the body's internal environment, namely the cells, tissues, organs and fluids (Clancy and McVicar 2002).

Maintenance of homeostasis depends primarily on providing an internal environment suitable for facilitating normal cellular function. Certain stimuli can result in alterations to the internal physical environment referred to as stressors, all of which have the ability to affect cellular function pathologically. Insults range from compromise to a specific cellular function, through to multi-organ failure and death. As a result, the internal environment is constantly changing or adapting; this is a direct result of physical, psychological and environmental stressors.

Extreme physiological sources include hypoxia and haemorrhaging, environmental sources include viruses and bacteria, radiation, and nutritional deficits, and psycho-social sources can be everyday minor stressors like job-related pressure, through to major life-altering events such as divorce and bereavement. Economical depression and social deprivation can also have prolonged and pathologic effects on homeostasis.

Homeostasis relies on a narrow margin for optimum fluid and electrolyte function; both of which are essential to normal function. Homeostasis is achieved by various organ systems working in unison to achieve a common goal: to maintain a constant state of optimum internal equilibrium.

The internal regulator, or controlling body, is the hypothalamus: a small and compact part of the brain working closely with the pituitary gland to regulate all organ systems via the release of hormones and hormonal precursors which activate several vital endocrine glands.

Imbalances resulting in either an excessive loss or retention of water, or an excess or deficiency of any of the main electrolytes can instigate a myriad of acute pathologies; clinical manifestations range from vomiting, diarrhoea and muscle cramps through to the development of life-threatening cardiac dysrhythmias such as ventricular tachycardia and torsade de pointe. Rectifying dysfunction and maintaining an internal environment compatible with normal cellular function are, therefore, essential elements of caring for every attending patient.

Normal perfusion

Cellular and organ perfusion is dependent on four components of the circulatory system.

The heart (the circulatory pump)

Heart rate and the force of contraction are under autonomic/involuntary control.

Sympathetic nerve fibres can:

- Increase both the rate and force of contractions
- Increase the blood pressure.

Parasympathetic fibres via the vagus nerve can:

- Reduce both the rate and force of contractions
- Reduce the blood pressure.

The stroke volume can also be increased resulting in an increased ejection fraction with each cardiac cycle. Both of these responses increase the flow of blood into the arteries and increase blood pressure.

Fluid volume (blood cells and plasma)

In the presence of normal physiology, the blood volume in the circulation directly equates to the preload received by the right side of the heart. According to Frank–Starling law, under normal conditions the greater the preload and stretch of myocardial fibres, the greater the force of myocardial contraction (see Box 2.1). Fluid components must be optimal to provide an adequate transportation medium for nutrients and oxygen. Red blood cells and their constituents are essential for oxygen transportation, a deficiency in carrier agents like haemaglobin (Hb), iron, or the red blood cells themselves, directly results in a reduced oxygen-carrying capacity. An increase in the thickness or viscosity of the blood will result in an increase in blood pressure and potential sludging or clotting of blood.

Box 2.1 Cardiac output (average under normal conditions)
• Stroke volume (SV) = 70mls • Heart rate (HR) = 70bpm • Cardiac output = SV × HR = 4900mls Cardiac output is the product of the heart rate multiplied by the stroke volume. It represents the efficiency with which the heart circulates the blood throughout the body.

An oxygenating system (the alveolar capillary interface)

Altered physiology within the pulmonary circuit may hinder the delivery of transported oxygen, or elimination of carbon dioxide. A classic acute example being a pulmonary embolus, and chronic compromise being impaired lung function due to chronic bronchitic conditions.

The containers (veins and arteries)

Large vessels such as the aorta need to expand when the heart ejects blood into them, therefore, they are composed of elastic fibres which can stretch and recoil. As blood travels through the arterial system, the arterial walls lose their elasticity which is replaced by smooth muscle. This change in composition allows the autonomic nervous system to directly influence the resistance arterial blood flow encounters by either, constricting or dilating the smooth muscle of arteries/arterioles. The higher the resistance, the higher the blood pressure. When arterial walls become diseased and thickened by athero-sclerosis, the blood flow may be compromised and the blood pressure is increased. The veins can expand and narrow; when veins expand, more blood can be stored and less blood returns to the heart for pumping into the arteries (a reduced preload). As a result, the heart receives less blood to pump, and the blood pressure is lowered. When veins narrow, there is a lower ability to house blood, excess blood is shunted back to the heart for pumping into the arteries and the heart ejects more blood into the systemic circulation, thus increasing the systemic pressure.

A derangement of any one of these components can impair perfusion and instigate physiological shock.

A patient who at rest appears well, demonstrates an excellent clinical example: once they mobilize, they become extremely short of breath, sweat profusely and become ashen grey or pale. Physiologically this patient may be demonstrating failure of all four of the aforementioned components of perfusion.

- First, although the heart may provide adequate perfusion at rest, once it is under increased pressure associated with exercise or movement, it may fail as an effective pump. There are many causes for this, which include previous myocardial infarction (MI), valve abnormalities and chronic hypertension leading to cardiac tissue remodelling (Vernooy et al. 2005).
- Second, the chronic disease state of hypertension can lead to activation of the renin angiotensin aldosterone axis (RAAS), exacerbating the clinical presentation (Clancy and McVicar 2002). The pathophysiological endpoint of this process is an alteration to the quality of heart muscle and blood osmolarity, resulting in the retention of fluid.
- Third, atherosclerosis and arteriosclerosis result not only in clogging of the arteries, but also continue the cycle of disease development by not supplying adequate perfusion to vital organs such as the heart and kidneys.
- Last, if the blood is not able to carry or deliver oxygen, the system fails.

Defining shock

Physiological shock can be defined as an inadequate circulatory volume to facilitate the oxygenation and nutritional needs of the body's cells; this internal insult is exacerbated by the subsequent insufficient removal of the waste products of cellular metabolism. Initially this can result in compensatory homeostatic responses, which aim to counteract the internally identified deficit or surplus of waste products. If internal equilibrium is not restored, the internal environment will become increasingly hypoxic and acidotic. This acidotic environment is not compatible with cellular function, initially resulting in cellular injury. Depending on the insult, this process can be instantaneous or have a gradual accumulative affect escalating from cell to tissue damage, and progressing to multi-organ failure.

The clinical application is that all serious illnesses have the potential to result in reduced cellular perfusion producing physiological shock.

What does compensation really mean?

The compensatory response phase aims to restore an adequate circulation. To achieve this there is a requirement for internal detection systems, which measure for fluctuations in certain essential substances within the blood: these are the chemo and baroreceptors. Fluctuations need to be closely monitored and acted upon, in a similar manner to a computer's cooling regulation system, in other words, when the internal computer components reach a certain temperature a sensor relays a message to a control mechanism which activates the fan to cool the hardware. Once a temperature below the sensory level is reached, the sensor stops sending the message and the control centre deactivates the fan. In reality, this is a continuous process, or feedback mechanism, affected by many variables, i.e., levels of activity.

Central control

Centrally located within the midbrain immediately above the pituitary gland, the hypothalamus can modify arterial blood pressure by instigating the fight or flight response (also called the sympathetic response). This is achieved by stimulating the lobes of the pituitary gland to release hormones, which affect certain endocrine organs, namely the adrenal glands to instigate localized change within the body, through the secretion of catecholamines into the central circulation (Figure 2.1).

Respiration and the chemoreceptors

The first sensors (receptors) involved in the feedback process are those involved in the maintenance of arterial blood gas homeostasis, these are the peripheral chemoreceptors located within major arteries; the chemoreceptors are stimulated by a rise in carbon dioxide levels and a fall in pH or oxygen levels within the blood. The respiratory centre receives the information as a nerve impulse from the chemoreceptors and uses this data to regulate breathing. Although both carbon dioxide and oxygen levels are monitored, due to the narrower physiological spectrum of carbon dioxide, it is this chemical, which, under normal conditions, initiates change. Oxygen levels, particularly hypoxaemia that provide a back-up mechanism, can become a primary focus for instigating change in the presence of a chronically altered physiology. This is referred to as the hypoxic drive, which is classically demonstrated by smokers suffering from chronic obstructive pulmonary disease (Chapter 9).

If there is a change in carbon dioxide levels outside the normal parameters (hyper/hypocapnia), the respiratory centre can transmit nerve impulses to the diaphragm and intercostal muscles causing inhalation and maintaining homeostasis through an increase, or decrease, in respiratory rate and depth. When sufficient air has entered the respiratory tracts, the stretch receptors (proprioceptors) in the alveoli and bronchioles detect full capacity and send inhibitory signals to the pneumotaxic centre to cause exhalation, and this feedback system is a continuous process. Initially if the insult is negligible, the compensatory phase may provide normal cellular perfusion by either blowing off or retaining carbon dioxide and subsequently increasing the level of circulating oxygen.

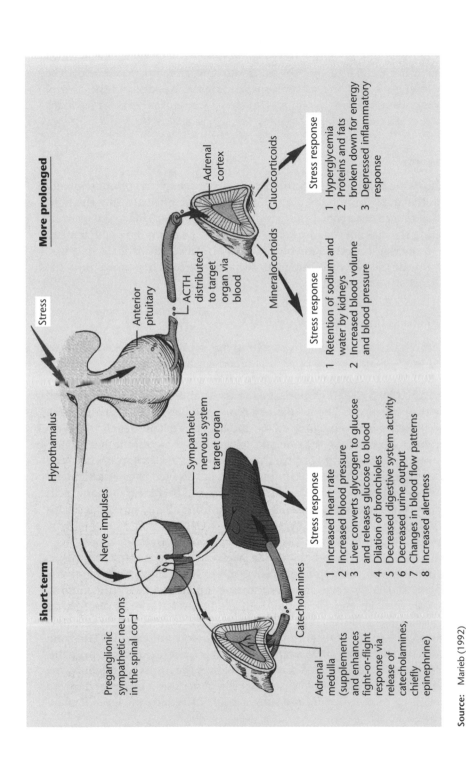

Source: Marieb (1992)

Figure 2.1 Role of the hypothalamus, adrenal medulla and adrenal cortex in the stress response (HRR)

Pressure regulation and the baroreceptors

Many internal mechanisms unify to maintain an adequate circulating volume: baroreceptors located in the aorta, carotid arteries and various organs detect changes in blood pressure. In a similar feedback mechanism to that of the chemoreceptors, nerve impulses are sent to the cardiac and vasomotor centres within the medulla oblongata and quick acting catecholamines such as adrenaline are released, initiating peripheral vasoconstriction and an increase in the force and rate of heart muscle contraction (Figure 2.1). The result is that blood is directed toward essential organs, this compensatory mechanism is referred to as central shunting, but is at the expense of other less essential organs such as the kidneys. The main function of the kidneys is to provide long-term regulation of blood pressure (the same principle as blood gas maintenance) by releasing erythropoietin, which initiates the formation of new red blood cells. The kidneys also influence vasoconstriction through the activation of the renin angiotensin system (RAS), and the reabsorption of sodium and electrolytes is achieved by the activation of mineralocorticoid aldosterone.

The RAS allows the kidneys to compensate for a loss in blood volume or decreases in blood pressure by increasing or decreasing the amount of urine that is produced. Water constitutes 96 per cent of urine, therefore, when the kidney makes more urine, the amount (volume) of blood that fills the arteries and veins decreases, and this lowers blood pressure. If urine production is curtailed, the amount of blood or fluid available to be re-absorbed into the circulation increases.

These adaptive responses will maintain the blood pressure within the normal range unless blood or fluid loss becomes so severe and protracted that the compensatory responses are overwhelmed.

Vital signs

Vital signs directly demonstrate the current physiological state of the patient, yet research has clearly demonstrated the inability of healthcare professionals to correctly interpret or act on recorded data. The most common mistake practitioners make is to underestimate the seriousness of the clinical data they have recorded, and this is of particular importance in relation to the blood pressure due to an over-reliance on this one component. Many clinicians fail to recognize the subtle signs of deterioration associated with shock until there is a dramatic decrease in the blood pressure (Tippins 2005). Box 2.2 demonstrates three clinical scenarios of patients experiencing differing levels of shock.

> **Box 2.2** Vital sign analysis
>
> *Case 1*: A 21-year-old male presents following an acute collapse with intense abdominal pain. Vital signs:
>
> - Respiratory rate 26
> - Pulse rate 79
> - Blood pressure 118/76
>
> *Case 2*: A 78-year-old female presents complaining of acute abdominal pain. Vital signs:
>
> - Respiratory rate 31
> - Pulse rate 109
> - Blood pressure 82/49
>
> *Case 3*: A 54-year-old male presents with a two-day history of increasing abdominal pain. Vital signs:
>
> - Respiratory rate 34
> - Pulse rate 142
> - Blood pressure 72/43

Vital sign analysis

- Case one demonstrates the subtle evidence of compensatory shock, which can be particularly difficult to distinguish in young normally fit individuals. In this instance, the normal expected vital signs may be a respiratory rate of 12, a pulse of 52 and a blood pressure of 115/70. In comparison, his vital signs on attendance reveal a significantly high respiratory rate, a pulse which is increased for his age range, particularly if recorded at rest, and a blood pressure within normal limits. This indicates that the internal compensatory mechanisms are maintaining homeostasis as the blood pressure is maintaining cellular perfusion. In short, this is referred to as the compensatory phase because the compensation is working (Figure 2.2).
- Case two highlights an increase in both respiratory and pulse rates. Although these increases are in conjunction with other internal mechanisms such as the RAAS, they still fail to maintain the blood pressure. Subsequently the patient's clinical condition becomes critical as they move into a decompensated or progressive phase of shock. The ability of the clinician to understand this terminology is paramount; decompensated meaning the internal compensatory

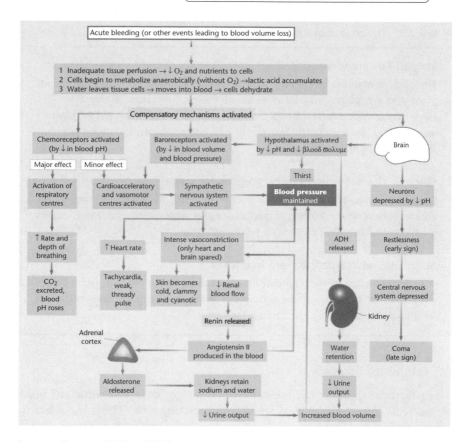

Source: Clancy and McVicar (2002)

Figure 2.2   Events and signs of hypovolaemic shock

mechanisms are not providing adequate perfusion and the shock is progressing.

- Case three demonstrates shock at the most frequently recognized stage (Box 2.3), unfortunately for the patient by this stage the internal environment has sustained potentially irreversible organ damage, and despite medical intervention, the patient's prognosis is poor. This stage of shock is referred to as irreversible or terminal shock, the next significant change in vital signs may reveal the failure or collapse of compensatory muscles and bradypnoea or bradycardia and respiratory/cardiac arrest will ensue.

Cases two and three demonstrate a decreased mean arterial pressure, with case three clearly exhibiting a pressure too low to maintain adequate cerebral oxygenation.

Box 2.3 The cycle of shock development

Stage I: The compensation stage

The body is able to compensate for the loss in circulation or tissue perfusion. Signs and symptoms may be minimal as the compensation is effective. This stage may provide adequate long-term compensation for healing to take place in minor insults. Because of the potency of internal regulators, the blood pressure may be normal or even elevated.

Stage II: The decompensatory/progressive stage

Despite the influence of compensatory mechanisms, the insult to homeostasis continues to progress, leading to inadequate vital organ perfusion. Unless urgent intervention is initiated, multiorgan failure will ensue.

Stage III: The irreversible/terminal stage

A prolonged state of reduced perfusion or a devastating insult to homeostasis will result in irreversible cellular damage involving major organs. Immediate and long-term compensatory mechanisms fail.

Possible misleading data

Many factors can affect the reliabilty of vital signs data and clinicians need to take this into consideration when interpretating data. These include any other internal mechanisms that initiate the fight or flight response. These mechanisms mimic the instigation of the compensatory phase of shock: pain, fear, anxiety and stimulants. In contrast, several commonly prescribed medications can inhibit the compensatory response: these include: beta-blockers and, to a certain extent, ACE inhibitors. These drugs because of their very nature directly block some of the internal compensatory responses and therefore impact on the validity of the data, therefore, it is absolutely vital to ascertain what medications a patient takes and their medical history before deciding their physiological status.

Mean arterial pressure

The mean arterial pressure (MAP) is the calculated pressure necessary to push blood through the systemic circulation and maintain essential organ perfusion. Keeping the MAP above 60mmHg will maintain cerebral perfusion, however, although this will prevent brain damage, it will not prevent renal failure as the arterial pressure is too low to adequately perfuse the renal system. Clinically this is evident by a reduced diuresis or oliguira (a classic late sign of shock). Most modern data recorders will calculate the MAP, despite this, clinicians should have a formula. How to calculate the MAP is demonstrated in Box 2.4.

Box 2.4 Calculating the mean arterial pressure

Systolic + (diastolic × 2) / by three

Case one (118/76): 118 + 76 × 2 = 270/3 = 90mmHg
Case two (82/49): 82 + 49 × 2 = 180/3 = 60mmHg
Case three (72/43): 72 + 43 × 2 = 158/3 = 52mmHg

Remember: a MAP of greater than 60 mmHg is needed to perfuse the organs of the average person. If the MAP remains consistantly around 60mmHg or continues to depreciate, major organ failure will develop.

Pulse pressure

The pulse pressure is the change in blood pressure seen during a contraction of the heart. As the left ventricle pumps blood into the systemic circulation, the pressure increases, as a general rule, an adequate stroke volume will provide an adequate pulse pressure. When confronted by a patient suspected of suffering shock, an estimate of their available blood flow can be made by calculating this pressure. At rest the average pulse pressure is around 40mmHg (120–80 = 40mmHg). This figure can be artificially increased by both with the aging process and chronic pathologies such as aortic stenosis that increase the pressure within the aorta. A decreasing pulse pressure i.e. < 30 mmHg, is a good indicator of a decrease in circulating volume and, therefore, an active loss of circulating fluid. This can be confirmed by observing for the compensatory rise in both the respiratory and pulse rates.

Defining the cause of shock

Defining the cause of shock will determine the focus of treatment, as the causative agent will need to be dealt with to combat the pathophysiological processes taking place. Shock is a progressive state and, therefore, early identification facilitates early intervention, which improves the patient's prognosis (Evans and Tippins 2005). A dramatic example is demonstrated in the management of meningitis. If left untreated until obvious signs like a haemorrhagic rash are evident, the long-term prognosis is poor.

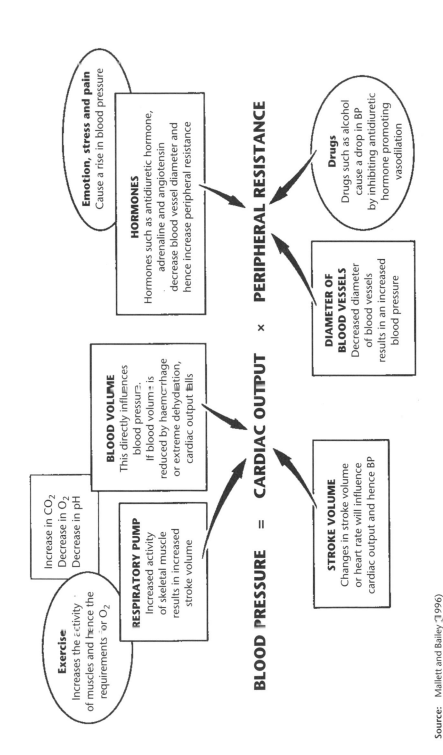

Emotion, stress and pain
Cause a rise in blood pressure

HORMONES
Hormones such as antidiuretic hormone, adrenaline and angiotensin decrease blood vessel diameter and hence increase peripheral resistance

Drugs
Drugs such as alcohol cause a drop in BP by inhibiting antidiuretic hormone promoting vasodilation

BLOOD VOLUME
This directly influences blood pressure.
If blood volume is reduced by haemorrhage or extreme dehydration, cardiac output falls

Increase in CO_2
Decrease in O_2
Decrease in pH

Exercise
Increases the activity of muscles and hence the requirements for O_2

RESPIRATORY PUMP
Increased activity of skeletal muscle results in increased stroke volume

STROKE VOLUME
Changes in stroke volume or heart rate will influence cardiac output and hence BP

DIAMETER OF BLOOD VESSELS
Decreased diameter of blood vessels results in an increased blood pressure

BLOOD PRESSURE   =   CARDIAC OUTPUT   ×   PERIPHERAL RESISTANCE

Source: Mallett and Bailey (1996)

Figure 2.3 Factors affecting changes in blood pressure

Types of shock

Five distinct categories of shock exist, although they share many similarities.

Box 2.5   Categories of shock

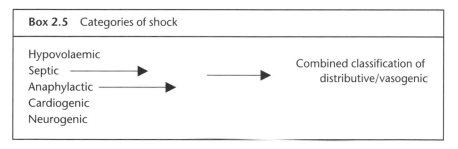

Hypovolaemic
Septic
Anaphylactic
Cardiogenic
Neurogenic

Combined classification of
distributive/vasogenic

Hypovolaemic shock

Hypovolaemia can be defined as an inadequate circulating fluid volume to facilitate cellular metabolism (Box 2.6). Hypovolaemia is the most frequent presentation of shock; this is because a low circulating fluid or blood volume (hypovolaemia) is the end point of many clinical conditions (Table 2.1).

Box 2.6   Assessing adequate circulation

When confronted by a patient who is potentially seriously ill, regardless of the setting, the clinician is expected to make a quick but factual assessment of the patient's circulation.

In many situations, clinicians become fixated with obtaining a blood pressure on a patient demonstrating obvious signs of inadequate circulation. These signs include:

- absent or weak radial pulse
- prolonged CRT
- decreased level of consciousness
- pale, cyanozed or mottled appearance.

This tick box approach to assessment can result in time wasted, which could have been utilized to treat the patient. Radial pulses provide an excellent indication of the patient's circulation.

Once the blood pressure has fallen < 90mmHg the radial pulse will become progressively weaker until it is lost. Small boluses of fluid can be titrated until the pulse is felt (usually 200–500mls). This is of particular importance in haemorrhagic shock where permissive hypotension has proved to be life-saving (Pepe 2003).

Table 2.1 Causes of hypovolaemia

Hypovolaemia secondary to haemorrhagic cause		Hypovolaemia secondary to fluid loss	
• External blood loss	• Penetrating trauma	• External fluid loss	• Burns
• Internal blood loss	• Blunt trauma	• Internal fluid loss	• Gastroenteritis
	• Ruptured aneurysm		(vomit-diarrhoea)

Hypovolaemia can be either a medical or surgical emergency, therefore, ascertaining the cause is essential to initiating appropriate treatment and referral.

Treatment of hypovolaemia (regardless of cause)

- Assess airway stability and administer high-flow oxygen.
- Gain IV access and commence fluid resuscitation (Box 2.6).
- If haemorrhagic, administer blood as soon as possible.
- Identify and treat cause (sepsis, cardiogenic, tamponade, tension pneumothorax).
- If the patient remains hypotensive, inotropic support, invasive monitoring and high dependency care are indicated.

Septic shock/systemic inflammatory response syndrome (SIRS)

Sepsis represents an uncontrolled inflammatory response to bacteraemia (pathogens in the blood), secondary to a severe infection from any source within the body and the subsequent failure of the internal defence mechanisms. The presence of certain bacteria within the blood results in extensive vasodilation and hypotension, as the circulating fluid is lost into the tissues.

SIRS represents a disease continuum (Box 2.7), a progressive and life-threatening clinical condition that can proliferate at an incredible rate; without early recognition and intervention the mortality rate can exceed 70 per cent.

There are an estimated 751,000 cases of severe sepsis/septic shock in the United States each year, similar to the number of deaths due to myocardial infarction (9.3 per cent of all deaths) accounting for in excess of 600 deaths per day (Guidet et al. 2005). Within the UK, the incidence of septicaemia is 7 in 1000 admissions to hospital, 20 per cent of these patients develop septic shock and 60–70 per cent of patients die due to septic shock development (Annane et al. 2004).

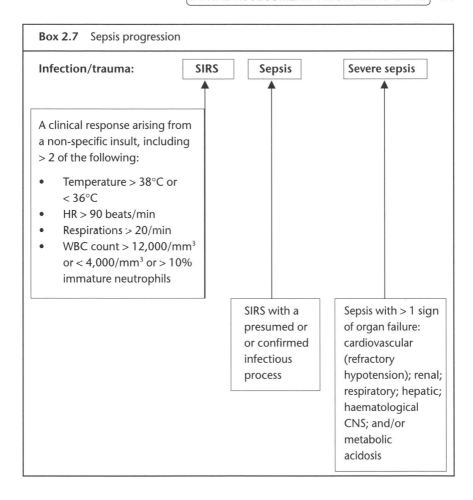

Box 2.7 Sepsis progression

Infection/trauma: → SIRS → Sepsis → Severe sepsis

A clinical response arising from a non-specific insult, including > 2 of the following:

- Temperature > 38°C or < 36°C
- HR > 90 beats/min
- Respirations > 20/min
- WBC count > 12,000/mm³ or < 4,000/mm³ or > 10% immature neutrophils

SIRS with a presumed or or confirmed infectious process

Sepsis with > 1 sign of organ failure: cardiovascular (refractory hypotension); renal; respiratory; hepatic; haematological CNS; and/or metabolic acidosis

Sepsis is usually seen in the very young or very old, those with weakened immune systems (through disease or compromise by immune-suppressing therapies), and those undergoing invasive treatments or surgery.

Treatment options

- Assess the patient's ability to maintain airway patency, early intubation and ventilation may be necessary to prevent respiratory failure.
- Fluid resuscitation may restore circulation; if hypovolaemia is refractory to fluid circulation, the early administration of inotropic drugs may reduce both future morbidity and mortality rates.
- The early identification of appropriate antibiotics is essential (Chapter 9).

Patients demonstrating septic shock require invasive monitoring in a high dependency area. The area of infection will need to be identified and samples sent for microculture and sensitivity (MC&S).

Anaphylactic shock

Anaphylaxis is a severe allergic reaction that is potentially fatal; it represents the clinical manifestation of a sequence of events resulting from a hypersensitivity reaction to an antigen. The prolific release of inflammatory mediators such as histamine result in the widespread symptoms summarized in Box 2.8.

Box 2.8 Signs and symptoms of anaphylaxis

- **Skin:** Vasodilation and capillary leakage causes urticaria and pruritus.
- **Respiratory:** Potential for complete airway obstruction due to laryngeal oedema (asphyxia). Over-secretion of mucus can result in bronchiole blockage and hypoxia. This is exacerbated by bronchiole smooth muscle constriction (bronchospasm).
- **Cardiovascular:** A complete collapse of the cardiovascular system is possible. Vasodilation/angio-oedema causes hypovolaemia, leading to a reduced CO.
- **Gastrointestinal:** Abdominal pain, nausea and vomiting and diarrhoea are potential findings.

Acute anaphylaxis is often poorly recognized and treated despite being both a common presentation and frequently, caused by clinicians via the administration of drugs (Evans and Tippins 2005). It is imperative that all clinicians are familiar with the assessment and treatment of anaphylaxis.

Treatment options

If either airway compromise or haemodynamic instability exists, the patient requires immediate administration of adrenaline via the subcutaneous or intramuscular route. The dose is 0.5ml increments of 1:1000 adrenaline, which is 10 times stronger than the dose given intravenously (IV) in cardiac arrest. The following sequence should be followed:

- Assess the airway and apply high-flow oxygen therapy (Chapter 9 identifies associated noises).
- Early referral to an anaesthetist may prove life-saving.

- If actual or potential airway compromise exists, administer adrenaline.
- Assess ability to breath (is wheezing present?).
- Assess circulation/systemic perfusion (Box 2.6): if inadequate, administer adrenaline and gain IV access.
- Secondary drugs include: anti-histamines, which will prevent further deterioration; steroids to reduce inflammation (although they take 4–6 hours to work); a beta-agonist to reduce smooth muscle contraction within the bronchioles; and IV fluids to restore circulation.

The Resuscitation Council (UK) has published specific guidelines on anaphylaxis (RCUK 2006).

Cardiogenic shock

Cardiogenic shock can be defined as a failure of the pumping ability of the heart, resulting in a compromised cardiac output and consequent hypotension. The signs and symptoms range from a shortness of breath associated with pulmonary odema as seen in exacerbations of left ventricular failure, through to complete compromise of the cardiac output resulting in cardiac arrest. The cause is predominately associated with myocardial infarction. Shock occurs due to a reduction in the quality and quantity of functioning heart muscle following a myocardial infarction. The physical signs and symptoms are dependent on how much muscle has been destroyed and which part of the heart has been affected. If the patient presentation is associated with bradycardia and hypotension, the prognosis is poor, as the heart rate fails to compensate for the reduced output (Chapter 3). Other causes include acute compromise to the heart's ability to function, including blunt trauma, tension pneumothorax (Chapter 5) and pericarditis.

Treatment options

- Assess stability and patency of the patient's airway, administer high-flow oxygen. Laying the patient flat may prove fatal due to orthopnoea.
- Assess for inadequate ventilation due to pulmonary oedema; the early administration of diuretics, nitrates and non-invasive ventilation may prove beneficial.
- Assess for inadequate circulation, gain IV access, when administering IV fluids, continuously monitor for signs of fluid overload, which could prove fatal.
- Identify and treat cardiac dysrhythmias and instigate continual cardiac monitoring.

- Early specialist referral and inotropic support/intra-aortic balloon counterpulsation may prove vital.

Neurogenic shock

Neurogenic shock is the least common form of shock; although a transient form of neurogenic shock is common to all emergency departments in the form of syncope, or faint, which has the same end result as neurogenic shock. The instigator is a loss of sympathetic tone or an increase in parasympathetic tone. Innervation of the sympathetic nervous system results in massive vasodilation, hypotension and bradycardia (bradycardia, warm peripheries and the instigating mechanism of injury are the cardinal signs). This response can be initiated by a primary trauma or stress that leads to widespread massive vasodilation. The associated pooling of blood leads to a reduced venous return and subsequent reduced cardiac output. Isolated intracranial injuries do not cause neurogenic shock, spinal cord injury, spinal shock and spinal anaesthetics are the most frequent instigators.

Treatment options

- The patient must be assessed for hypovolaemia due to other causes such as haemorrhage first.
- If a head injury is present, be particularly cautious of airway instability.
- IV access and fluid administration may not increase circulating volume.
- The judicious use of vasopressors and anticholinergics such as atropine are recommended (American College of Surgeons 2004). These drugs counteract the innervation of the sympathetic nervous system.

Table 2.2 Physical signs synonymous with all forms of shock

Physical signs	Internal instigators
• Increase in respiratory rate and depth, cyanosis	• ↑ CO_2 or ↓ O_2 levels
• Normally tachycardia – also bradycardia	• Adrenaline/noradrenaline release
• Hypotension	• Loss of circulating volume
• Sweating – altered body temperature	• Adrenaline secretion
• Pale, cold, clammy skin	• Adrenaline secretion
• Decreased urine output	• Reduced renal blood supply
• Altered levels of consciousness	• Cerebral hypoxia/hypercapnia
• Thirst	• Release of anti-diuretic hormone/ vasopressin (ADH)

Cyanosis

Cyanosis is defined as a blue discoloration of the skin indicating excessive amounts of deoxygenated haemoglobin in the arterial vessels. Peripheral cyanosis found on the fingertips can indicate an impairment of local blood supply and can be instigated by cold weather and superficial vasoconstriction. It is also synonymous with chronic disease states leading to reduced oxygenation, i.e., heart failure. When centrally located, cyanosis is life-threatening, indicating failure of the heart and lungs to provide adequate oxygenation.

When initially assessing a patient, the obvious signs and symptoms of shock are not always easily apparent, the whole picture needs to be examined, including the presenting history.

Initial assessment

The following clinical scenario represents an everyday patient presentation. Scenario one demonstrates the standard structured approach that all ED nurses need to follow when initially assessing a patient. The assessment is structured using the ABCDE format endorsed by the internationally recognized advanced trauma life support and advanced life support (ATLS/ALS) courses (Box 2.10). This structure enables the practitioner to undertake an instantaneous, thorough and safe physical assessment of the patient's immediate needs, the focal point being the early recognition of serious illness and the subsequent correct prioritization of resources.

There are numerous assessment models, or mnemonics, currently adapted to suit the needs of acutely ill patients and clinical practice. The Resuscitation Council in the United Kingdom (RCUK, 2006) recommends the universal adoption of the ABCDE structure (see Box 2.10), where each component addresses a separate, but intrinsically linked body component.

Box 2.9 Level of consciousness

A = Alert
V = Responds to a verbal stimulus
P = Responds to a painful stimulus
U = Unresponsive

Box 2.10 ABCDE mnemonic

A = Airway and cervical spine immobilization
B = Breathing and ventilation
C = Circulation and haemorrhage control
D = Disability and neurological assessment
E = Exposure and environment

Scenario 2.1   Hypovolaemic shock

Hilda Jones, a 79-year-old Caucasian female, attends your emergency department with a vague history of lethargy and collapse. Her neighbour who visits each morning found her on the floor.

   She is able to complete a sentence although her mouth and mucous membranes appear very dry. Her respiratory rate is regular, bi-laterally shallow and recorded as 21. There are no signs of central or peripheral cyanosis. Her radial pulse is weak, regular and recorded as 117bpm, this is in conjunction with a distal capillary refill time of three seconds. The patient appears frightened, as she can't remember how or why she collapsed. She is pale, but not sweaty and clammy.

   She obeys commands but isn't orientated to time and place, her AVPU score is A (Box 2.9). Her pupils are equal, reactive to light and sized as 4mm (Chapter 8).

   She feels cold to touch both at a peripheral and central level. There are several bruises and some minor abrasions to both her hips and legs, which, due to discoloration appear to be old, and from previous injuries.

   She hasn't been well over the last week due to experiencing diarrhoea and vomiting.

   The patient has no known medical history or allergies.

Analysis of Scenario 2.1

D *Data* (scientific facts): from the primary data gathered, the patient demonstrates early signs of shock development. There is no initial evidence of actual airway compromise although the respiratory rate is slightly raised, possibly demonstrating respiratory compensation for an inadequate circulation, confirmed by the reduced CRT, tachycardia and a weak distal pulse, all indicative of shock development (Box 2.11). A blood pressure will be recorded to confirm the presence of hypovolaemia. If the patient has a near normal blood pressure, the compensation is working, if the pressure is reduced, the patient demonstrates progressive or decompensated shock.

   Mrs Jones appears dry, indicating a possible reduction in circulating volume or an electrolyte imbalance. There are no obvious physical deformities and neurologically Mrs Jones is alert and responding appropriately to stimuli. Although the patient feels cold, this is not a reliable indicator of body temperature particularly in the elderly and a central temperature should be recorded.

   An in-depth medical history will be needed to identify the possibility of drug toxicity, and a blood analysis may identify an electrolyte imbalance or a blood abnormality such as anaemia. The patient will require continual cardiac monitoring in conjunction with a 12-lead electrocardiogram (ECG).

Box 2.11 Capillary refill time (CRT)

The recording of a CRT in addition to a radial pulse is an excellent indicator of peripheral perfusion.

The patient's nail bed is compressed for five seconds with sufficient pressure to cause blanching. Once pressure is released, the nail bed should be engorged with blood and return to normal.

- In adults a CRT of two seconds or less will indicate good peripheral perfusion.
- A prolonged CRT should be interpreted in conjunction with other circulatory parameters, such as pulse rate, blood pressure, and conscious level (RCUK 2006).

This figure can be prolonged in the elderly, in a cold environment, and in the presence of poor ambient lighting or circulation-based anomalies such as Raynaud's Phenomenon.

E *Emotions* (intuition): when an elderly patient attends with a collapse of unknown origin, the possibility of the cause being cardiovascular in origin and potentially serious is high. This is closely followed by infection and drug toxicity (usually iatrogenic in cause). It is commonly stated by experienced practitioners that they can sense when a patient is unwell, or about to deteriorate (Tippins 2005).

In fact, several clinical signs will be evident at an early stage and although the practitioner may feel the basis for their initial priority is based on gut feelings or intuition, it could be argued that in contrast they have formulated their initial plan through unconsciously recognizing clinical signs and indicators of serious illness from the physical presentation and history which are clearly apparent with experience. The experienced clinician will assign the patient to a high dependency area and prioritize them accordingly, thereby expediting the patient's treatment and care.

A *Advantages*: patients presenting with collapse 'query cause' are a common presentation to all emergency staff. This presentation should be taken extremely seriously, particularly in the elderly patient as the likelihood of the collapse being related to a serious pathology is high and immediate data collection is required to negate the possibility of a cardiac dysrhythmia, severe infection, and hypo/hyperglycaemia. As with all potentially serious presentations, the clinician should commence supplementary oxygen therapy (potentially a life-saving intervention in some pathologies). An oxygen saturation probe should be used to ascertain the patient's baseline oxygenation status although this can be an unreliable test and obtaining an arterial blood gas would be more comprehensive although more invasive. Early intravenous access and the requisition of relevant blood tests will not only expedite care but also play a vital role in the patient's diagnosis and ongoing treatment plan. Intravenous fluids will be needed to rehydrate the patient: these should be commenced with caution as the patient may have underpinning heart failure. Other vital signs should be recorded along with the patient's postural blood pressure; a postural drop may indicate a cause of collapse, in elderly patients iatrogenic-induced postural hypotension is a common presentation (Box 2.12).

Box 2.12 Recording postural blood pressures

Rationale: Under normal conditions autonomic reflexes stabilize an individual's blood pressure from the lying to sitting/standing positions. This can be seen as the initiation of quick response mediators that result in peripheral vasoconstriction and shunting of blood into the main circulation.

When there is an established loss of circulating volume in the peripheries, this mechanism fails and a fall in blood pressure results, therefore, the recording of a postural blood pressure is an excellent eliminative tool to the practitioner suspecting a patient to be in the early stages of shock.

Example of a patient experiencing reduced circulating volume:

* Lying B/P 105/70 H/R 90
* Sitting B/P 85/58, H/R 115

A positive result is achieved if the patient's blood pressure demonstrates a systolic drop of > 20mmHg from laying to standing, or > 15mmHg from laying to sitting, although the differential may be slightly less, and this is offset by dangling the patient's legs over the trolley and the reduction in risk potential.

Rises in heart rate exceeding 20bpm, or a diastolic drop exceeding 10mmHg are also positive indicators. If circumstances allow, lay the patient supine for five minutes, record a blood pressure and heart rate, then assist them to sit up, allow one–three minutes, then record vital signs with the patient's legs dangling over the side of the trolley.

Be aware of the possibility that your patient may become acutely unwell and document any changes to their initial assessment findings.

D *Disadvantages* (**differential diagnosis**): the presentation of a collapse of unknown origin is an excellent example of how practitioners need to negate serious life-threatening presentations before moving on to less complex or insidious pathology. Taking an exact history is paramount, in this case the patient presents with acute dehydration secondary to diarrhoea and vomiting which has left her unable to eat or drink appropriately for the last week. Dehydration can affect any individual although the elderly, very young and those in a chronically weakened state experience increased rates of hospitalization and mortality.

When confronted with a patient who has experienced an acute collapse, the possibility of a cardiac/respiratory arrest or other significant life-threatening emergency needs to be negated immediately. This is achieved through the use of a structured approach (ABCDE). This risk assessment is a crucial component of providing excellence in care.

This initial scenario identifies the importance of a timely, yet comprehensive initial and ongoing assessment. The identification of the early warning signs of developing shock is what differentiates the novice and experienced practitioner. The following chapters will highlight various pathologies affecting specific internal body systems.

3 Acute cardiac emergencies: implications in clinical practice

Cliff Evans

Introduction

Cardiac emergencies are frequent and potentially life-threatening conditions that present to all acute emergency areas. The causes include congenital abnormalities, electrolyte disturbances and the general wear and tear associated with aging.

The majority of patient presentations share a common disease process, the endpoint being an ischaemic and diseased heart. Once established, this heart disease is progressive, debilitating and culminates in a direct reduction to the length and quality of the individual's life. Heart disease clinically manifests in several ways including: shortness of breath particularly on exertion, ankle oedema, physical collapse and cardiac arrest. When the heart eventually becomes acutely compromised or ischaemic, the physical manifestation the patient demonstrates is usually chest pain.

Clinicians working within emergency care are predominantly the initial contact point for patients presenting with acute chest pain. The ability of the clinician to make a quick, but prioritized assessment of the patient can prove, first, to be life-saving and, second, to have a large impact on the quality of the patient's future life. The initial professional responsibility when assessing patients attending with chest pain is, therefore, vast, as this phase of their care is paramount to the patient's prognosis.

This chapter commences with an overview of coronary heart disease (CHD) and the acute coronary syndromes (ACS). The reader will then be introduced to the electrocardiographic changes associated with diseases of the heart. Scenarios will be used to demonstrate common clinical findings and shed light on some of the many potential cardiac pathologies, enabling practitioners to gain an insight into many potential patient presentations.

The chapter concludes with a brief overview of the recently introduced guidelines on advanced life support and how they impact on the clinician's clinical decision-making (RCUK 2006).

Prevalence

Heart and circulatory disease are the biggest killers in both the United States and the United Kingdom. In 2002, cardiovascular disease (CVD) caused 39 per cent of deaths in the UK: around 238,000 people. A similar percentage of deaths can be found within the USA where 71 million American adults demonstrate an established CVD (AHA 2006).

The mortality rates, however, represent only the tip of the iceberg, the associated morbidity is enormous with varying degrees of chronic illness and incapacity. The annual cost to the individual, society and healthcare is vast. The healthcare cost is set to increase as precipitating factors like morbid obesity and associated illnesses, such as Type 2 diabetes and hypertension, escalate each year (BHF 2005). An example of the impact CVD is placing on the NHS is demonstrated by the reliance on the pharmaceutical industry for both preventative medicines, and medicines for chronic and acute episodes of the disease process. During 2003, 180 million prescriptions within the UK were written for diseases of the circulatory system, with the cost for lipid lowering drugs alone exceeding £713 million per year, and this figure is set to increase dramatically as clinicians try to meet national and international health targets (BHF 2005).

Coronary heart disease represents the majority of emergency presentations of CVD, causing approximately one in five deaths in men, and one in six deaths in women: approximately 117,000 deaths per year in the UK (BHF 2005). Although death rates for CHD have been falling rapidly in the UK since the late 1970s, they are still among the highest in Western Europe (BHF 2005). There is considerable variation in the development of CHD across the UK. Death rates are higher in Scotland than the south of England, in manual workers than in non-manual workers, and in certain ethnic groups. These death rates are largely preventable and, therefore, the subject of several national and international guidelines including the DoH's National Service Framework (NSf) for CHD (DoH 2000) which sets specific targets to reduce morbidity and mortality rates, and the European Society for Cardiology's evaluation of the effectiveness of acute treatment options (ESC 2005).

Pathophysiology

CHD and CVD relate to pathophysiological changes that take place within the circulatory system (the reader is referred to Saladin (2005) for an in-depth overview of the heart's anatomy and physiology). In the case of CHD, this process takes place within the coronary arteries affecting the delivery of blood to the heart. There are two interrelated disease processes leading to CHD.

Arteriosclerosis occurs as part of the aging process in which arterial walls gradually become ridged, inelastic and thickened due to the deposition of fibrous tissue. The end effect of thickened and inelastic vessels is an increase in blood pressure and an inability to alter lumen size (Chapter 2). This renders the vessel at an increased risk of rupture or occlusion, and a prime example is demonstrated by aortic stenosis. Atherosclerosis is the term used to describe the deposition of lipid and cholesterol-rich atheromatous plaques within the arterial walls. Over time the inner lumen becomes increasingly clogged, resulting in a reduced distal blood flow. These atheromatous plaques have a serious risk of dislodgement, leading to thrombus formation in a narrower part of the lumen and complete distal occlusion.

Several theories exist to the origin of atheromatous plaques, and one is that fat is the ultimate source of potential energy, therefore it is stored throughout the body for times of need, and there may be a genetic predisposition exacerbating this phenomena. Due to modern methods of farming and food production, in addition to growing wealth and an all-year-round availability of food, this potential period of starvation is never realized, resulting in the excessive accumulation of fatty deposits within the arteries. It is accepted that if a surplus amount of fat is consumed within the diet and not utilized through energy requirements (exercise), then it is deposited not only in visible subcutaneous areas, but also within the walls of the arteries. This process is insidious with studies identifying cholesterol deposits within the arteries as early as the teenage years (DoH 2000). Box 3.1 identifies some of the predisposing factors to the development of atherosclerosis and CHD.

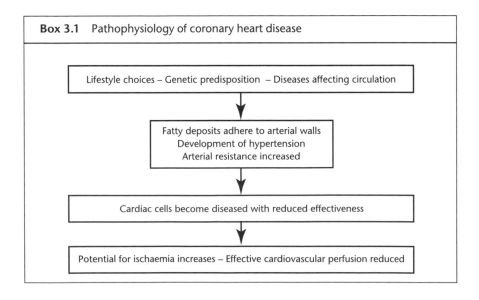

Box 3.1 Pathophysiology of coronary heart disease

Lifestyle choices – Genetic predisposition – Diseases affecting circulation

Fatty deposits adhere to arterial walls
Development of hypertension
Arterial resistance increased

Cardiac cells become diseased with reduced effectiveness

Potential for ischaemia increases – Effective cardiovascular perfusion reduced

As previously stated, many cardiac conditions share a common cause or alteration to normal coronary perfusion and function: collectively these are termed the acute coronary syndromes (ACS).

Acute coronary syndromes

The acute coronary syndromes reflect a disease continuum, comprising three distinct stages of disease progression. These range from unstable angina, with episodes of ischaemic pain at rest; non-ST elevated myocardial infarction (NSTEMI), where there has been limited damage to the heart muscle; and culminating in infarctions, which extend through the full thickness of the heart muscle demonstrating the classic ECG changes synonymous with acute myocardial infarction (STEMI) (Box 3.2).

Although this is a progressive illness, a patient can attend with an acute STEMI despite having no history of angina or a formal diagnosis of major instigating factors, i.e., hypertension.

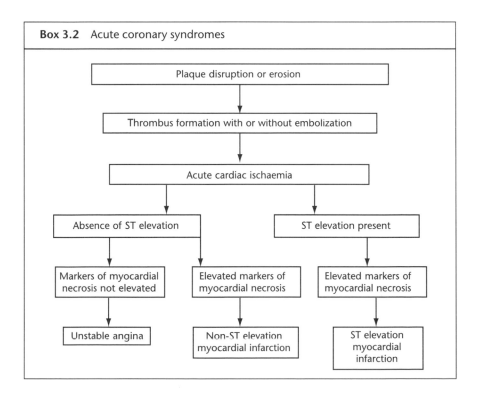

Box 3.2 Acute coronary syndromes

Plaque disruption or erosion

Thrombus formation with or without embolization

Acute cardiac ischaemia

Absence of ST elevation

ST elevation present

Markers of myocardial necrosis not elevated

Elevated markers of myocardial necrosis

Elevated markers of myocardial necrosis

Unstable angina

Non-ST elevation myocardial infarction

ST elevation myocardial infarction

Unstable angina

Theoretically there is no universally accepted definition for unstable angina. Clinically it manifests with the individual experiencing the type of chest pain associated with angina, at rest rather than on exertion, with increased severity or prolongation and cardiac-related chest pain in an individual previously undiagnosed with angina.

Unstable angina, NSTEMI and STEMI are closely related, with clinical presentations that may be indistinguishable. Their division centres on whether the ischaemic episode is severe enough to cause damage or death to the heart muscle. If death has occurred, subsequent biochemistry examination will provide evidence of a rise in enzymes that are released into the blood stream when heart muscle dies. These cardiac enzymes or markers of myocardial necrosis initially centre on one particular enzyme called troponin. Troponin serum levels increase within 3–12 hours from the onset of chest pain, and peak at 24–48 hours, returning to baseline over 5–14 days (Ghuran et al. 2003).

Non-ST elevated myocardial infarction (NSTEMI)

If the instigating thrombus disperses before complete distal tissue ischaemia and necrosis have occurred, the infarction will not extend completely through the heart muscle, subsequently only a localized area of myocardium, usually deep within the heart will be affected. As the main part of musculature which conducts electricity is left unscathed, this will not, therefore, be associated

Table 3.1 Clinical signs, symptoms and risk factors associated with AMI

Clinical signs	Risk factors
• Chest pain – commonly central and radiating into the neck, arms or jaw.	• Previous AMI
	• Diabetes mellitus
• Sweaty clammy or ashen grey appearance	• Obesity
	• Genetic pre-disposition (Afro-Caribbeans/
• Nausea or vomiting	Asians)
• Chest pain can be masked by diabetic neuropathy	• Smoking
	• Stimulant use (cocaine)
• Sudden collapse of unknown cause	• Family history of CHD/CVD
• Shortness of breath/Dyspnoea	• Sedentary lifestyle
• Crushing sensation to central chest	• Hypertension
	• Hypercholesterolaemia/lipidaemia

with ST elevation and Q wave formation. These presentations have the potential to re-infarct as the atherosclerotic plaque is disrupted and may prompt further thrombus formation through the aggregation of platelets (thrombocytes). Ischaemic damage results in scar tissue formation, this is fibrous, inelastic and causes a permanent decrease in the contractility and ejection potential of the heart.

The diagnosis of unstable angina or NSTEMI necessitates urgent hospital admission and cardiac monitoring (Box 3.4). The clinical history, physical presentation, 12-lead electrocardiography and measurement of cardiac enzyme concentrations within the blood are the essential diagnostic tools.

ST elevated myocardial infarction (STEMI)

STEMI can be defined as the death or necrosis of part of the myocardium due to the complete cessation of the local blood supply causing inadequate cellular oxygenation (Figure 3.1). The primary cause is the rupture of atheromatous deposits within the coronary arteries, and the subsequent formation of a clot

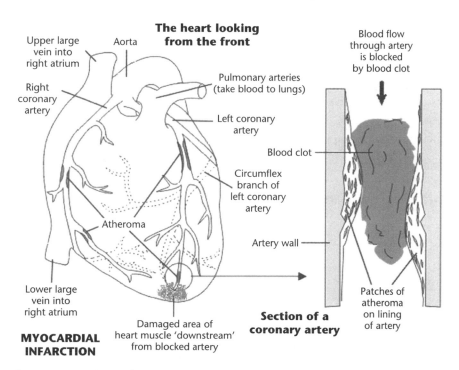

Source: www.patient.co.uk (Reproduced with permission)

Figure 3.1   What happens when you have a myocardial infarction?

(thrombus). The infarction can extend from the endocardium to epicardium resulting in severe cardiac dysfunction, and the characteristic development of the ECG changes of ST elevation and later Q wave formation.

Thirty-three per cent of males and 25 per cent of females die instantaneously, post-myocardial infarction 50 per cent of patients will go on to die within 30 days of the event. Those who survive will develop varying degrees of heart failure.

Since the introduction of the NSF in March 2000, treatment times for patients attending with cardiac disease have been decreasing. In 2003, 75 per cent of patients eligible for thrombolysis were treated within 20 minutes of arrival, more than double for the same period in 2000 (MINAP 2004).

When a patient presents to the ED with an acute onset of chest pain, it is usually because previous attempts to relieve the pain have failed; these may have included the administration of GTN (nitrates) or analgesics. The assessment process needs to negate a possible STEMI with the emphasis on urgency – as time is muscle.

Box 3.3 The three stages of AMI development

- **Ischaemic** – tissue damage caused by a lack of oxygen. Early administration of O_2 therapy can salvage the potential damage.
- **Injury** – greater degree of damage, but still salvageable with the early instigation of treatment.
- **Infarction** – necrotic/dead tissue depending on timescale damage can be limited or cardiac arrest prevented.

Clinicians can have a direct positive effect on their patient's long-term outcomes by acting quickly and efficiently.

Initial assessment

The initial diagnosis and subsequent treatment of AMI are currently based on the patient meeting two of the three possible initial diagnostic criteria, first, a physical presentation demonstrating the clinical signs of ischaemic heart disease (Table 3.1). Second, electrocardiogram (ECG) changes synonymous with the identification of a new left bundle branch block (LBBB); STEMI (this includes S-T segment elevation in ECG leads that would normally view a positive electric current); or S-T segment depression in leads that view the anterior aspect of the heart which can indicate a potential mirror image of S T elevation in the posterior region (reciprocal changes) (Table 3.2). The third diagnostic factor relates to enzymatic changes, due to the related time-scale needed to obtain these results they traditionally had no role in the initial working

Table 3.2   Area of infarction

Area of Infarction	ECG leads
Inferior	II, III, aVF
Inferiolateral	II, III, aVF, V5, V6
	Sometimes I and aVL
Inferioseptal	II, III, aVF, V1, V2, V3
Anterior	VI–V4, sometimes V5
Anterioseptal	V1, V2, V3
Anteriolateral	I, aVL V1–V6
Lateral	I, aVL V5, V6
Posterior	VI–V3 show reciprocal changes (ST – depression)
	Often associated with inferior infarction

Box 3.4   High acute risk factors for progression to myocardial infarction or death

Patients meeting any of these criteria should undergo coronary angiography within 48 hours:

- Recurrent chest pain at rest.
- Dynamic ST-segment changes: ST-segment depression > 0.1 mV or transient (< 30mins) ST-segment elevation > 0.1 mV.
- Elevated Troponin-I, Troponin-T, or CK-MB levels.
- Haemodynamic instability within the observation period.
- Major arrhythmias (ventricular tachycardia, ventricular fibrillation).
- Early post-infarction unstable angina.
- Diabetes mellitus.

---

diagnosis (ESC, 2005). Recent advances in both the accessibility of point of care diagnostic tests and their reliability, may result in enzymatic changes playing a larger role in the initial management phase.

Patients attending with NSTEMI need to be assessed or classified for their potential risk of an acute thrombotic episode (ESC 2005). Box 3.4 demonstrates the characteristics associated with a high risk potential for rapid progression to myocardial infarction or death.

Assessing the ECG

Emergency presentations related to either an alteration of the normal electrodynamics of the heart, or other disease processes that result in a derangement of cardiac function, are an everyday occurrence within emergency care. Clinicians working within the acute sector, therefore, require a solid foundational knowledge of both the theory and clinical application of skills within this area. The electrocardiogram (ECG) is one principal diagnostic tool the clinician can use to determine the presenting pathology and any subsequent treatment. The clinician's ability to understand and accurately interpret an ECG is essential to the patient's initial management and subsequent prognosis. This ability to record, interpret and act on the findings of an ECG is not an overnight achievement, therefore, the following guide to ECG analysis is presented in a format that practitioners can work through at their own pace, and ultimately develop clinical competence and confidence. In addition, the guide provides an aide-mémoire to certain 'problem' presentations, and a reference point for clinicians at work.

The first five stages provide a systematic approach to the essentials of basic rhythm interpretation, and are a good starting point for less experienced practitioners.

The systematic approach is based on the practitioner following a set sequence of questions that combine to build a complete picture of the underpinning cardiac conduction sequence. Through identifying the origin and stability of the presenting rhythm, the practitioner can adeptly progress to establish many common pathologies.

ECG recognition: the basics

The clinician will need to understand both the anatomy of the heart and the physiology of the cardiac cycle to enable them to gain understanding of the electrophysiological component of heart function. The reader is referred to Houghton and Gray (2003) for a comprehensive and in-depth overview of the electrophysiology of the heart.

Historically the main waveforms present on an ECG are the P, Q, R, S, T and U waves (Figure 3.2). These waveforms either represent the electrical discharging within the heart (depolarization) or electrical recharging (repolarization).

The ECG enables the clinician to calculate how long, in seconds, each part of the cardiac cycle lasts. The paper moves through the machine at a constant rate of 25mm/second, therefore by measuring the width of a wave the viewer can determine the duration of the event (Figure 3.2).

Is the rhythm regular?

Use a blank piece of paper and identify a significant point on the ECG such as an R wave (a rhythm strip or lead II are the best options). Identify and mark at

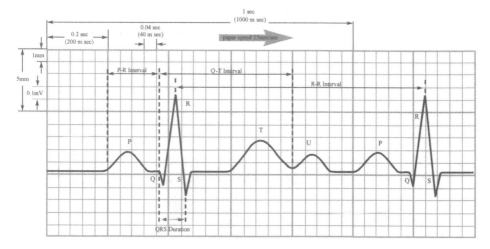

Figure 3.2   Electrical discharges within the heart (C. Evans, G. White)

Table 3.3   The correlation between electrophysiology and ECG waveforms

Heart function	ECG waveform
• Atrial systole/depolarization	• P Wave
• Atrial systole to commencement of ventricular activity	• PR interval
• Ventricular systole/depolarization	• QRS complex
• Endpoint of ventricular systole pre-repolarization	• ST segment
• Ventricular diastole/repolarization	• T wave
• Length between ventricular activity de/repolarization	• QT interval
• Possible interventricular septal repolarization	• U wave

least three consecutive R waves, move the paper along, if the points corre-
spond with proceeding R waves, the rhythm is regular, if the points do not
coincide, the rate is irregular.

The use of a prolonged rhythm strip is especially useful in the detection of
blocks and occasional dysrhythmias.

Calculate the ventricular/atrial rates

Counting the large boxes between two R waves (ventricular activity) and dividing this number into 300 determines the ventricular rate per minute.

Counting the large boxes between two P waves (atrial activity) and dividing this number into 300 determines the atrial rate per minute.

Figure 3.2 demonstrates that each small square = 0.04 seconds, one large square = 0.2 seconds. Therefore 5 large squares = 1 second, consequently 300 large squares = one minute. Thus, by dividing by 300 the rate over one minute is established.

If you have established the rate to be irregular, measure the large squares between the R waves that are the closest together and then the R waves which are furthest away from each other; this will ascertain the two extremes of the rate.

This is very useful in establishing the ventricular response in dysrhythmias such as atrial fibrillation or complete heart block.

Is atrial activity present and is there a relationship with QRS complexes?

For example, is every P wave followed by a QRS complex, or is there an underlying dysrhythmia or block?

If no P waves are visible, there are two potential causes:

1   No coordinated atrial activity present and therefore no P waves.
2   P waves are present but not obvious, i.e., obscured by a larger waveform.

What is the P-R interval?

Count the number of small squares between a P and R wave.

This is normally between 3–5 small squares (Figure 3.2).

This is very important for establishing heart blocks. For example, if the P-R interval is prolonged, this signifies a delay in the conduction sequence. In contrast, if the P-R interval is short, an underlying pathology like the Wolff-Parkinson-White syndrome may be present.

Is the QRS complex width normal?

Ventricular conduction is reflected by the QRS complex and is larger than the P wave, which represents the atrial contraction. This is due to two factors: first, the relative size of the ventricles in comparison to the atria and, second, the anatomical origin of the electrical stimulus.

The length of the QRS complex should not exceed 0.12 seconds, represented by three small squares on the ECG; otherwise it is considered to be abnormally wide, signifying a delay in ventricular conduction.

A common cause of a wide QRS complex is an extra beat (ectopic = early, escape = late) arising from a ventricular focus (Figure 3.3).

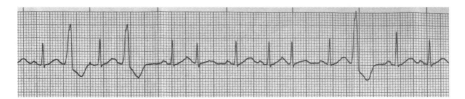

Figure 3.3 Premature ventricular contraction (ectopic)

Determining a possible infarction

The characteristic ECG changes associated with ischaemic events or myocardial infarction are best seen in the ECG leads that record that particular area (Table 3.2).

Familiarity with the areas of myocardium represented by each ECG lead therefore enables the viewer to visualize not only the localization, but also the extent of infarction.

The four limb leads are combined to provide six views of the heart. This is in addition to the six chest leads which coalesce to create a fairly comprehensive view of the electrical conduction of the heart.

The limb leads view the heart from the side, aVR the right side, aVL the left side and aVF upward from the angle of the feet.

Leads II, III and aVF represent the inferior surface of the heart. Chest leads VI–V4 record from the anterior surface of the heart. The lateral border of the heart is represented in leads I and aVL, and chest leads V5 and V6. The interventricular septum is represented in leads VI, V2 and V3.

Reciprocal changes can be viewed in opposing leads, for example, if the ST segment elevation associated with AMI is present in the anterior leads, the viewer will often see S-T depression in the inferior leads. This method of analysis is of particular importance when assessing for a posterior infarction, as the posterior view is not demonstrated in a normal 12-lead ECG. The clinician will need to assess the anterior leads (V2–4) for evidence of S-T depression or T wave inversion. In conjunction with tall R waves, this may represent reciprocal changes for ST elevation in the posterior leads. Box 3.5 demonstrates the recording of the 15-lead ECG, which can provide the clinician with a far better view of the heart.

Analyse chest leads V1–V6

Start at lead V1 and work through to lead V6 (right to left), identify any areas demonstrating evidence of S-T segment elevation, or T wave inversion/depression.

Box 3.5 Recording a 15 lead ECG

The ability to record a 15-lead ECG is an advanced skill the clinician can utilize to obtain a greater in-depth view of the heart.

The 15-lead ECG incorporates V4R and has the bonus of two posterior leads. These additional views are demonstrated at the expense of V4, V5 and V6.

- All leads continue on the horizontal plane (5th intercostal space).
- V4 is placed in the same anatomical site although to the right of the sternum.
- V5 becomes V8 and is placed mid-scapular.
- V6 becomes V9 by being placed to the right of V8 and left to the spine (paraspinal).

If ST elevation is identified, look for reciprocal changes (imagine a mirror image) in leads that look at the heart from another view, i.e., if ST elevation is identified in leads V2–V4, then look for reciprocal S-T depression in the inferior leads II, III and aVF.

Once ST elevation is identified, refer to other leads that also reflect the identified area of potential infarction i.e. if ST elevation is identified in the lateral chest leads V5 V6, then assess the other lateral chest leads, i.e., leads 1 and aVL.

Inferior AMI and associated complications

There is a high association between inferior AMI and the development of serious complications including profound hypovolaemia and conduction disturbances. If you identify ST-elevation in leads II, III or aVF, you will need to establish whether the right ventricle is involved, the rationale being that the patient is at high risk of developing cardiogenic shock due to the failure of the right ventricle to provide an adequate filling pressure (through the lungs) to the left ventricle (Frank–Starling law). This possibility can be identified by recording a right-sided ECG (Houghton and Gray 2003). Traditionally the practitioner removes all chest leads and applies them to the same anatomical position on the right of the chest. A quick method can be to only replace lead V4 from the left to the same anatomical place on the right. This position is now referred to as V4R. If ST elevation is present, the patient will require fluid resuscitation before reperfusion therapy commences (please refer to your local department guidelines). Remember to clearly document this change.

Summarize your findings

State your initial findings using the systematic approach to add structure to your working diagnosis. Now critically analyse the results in conjunction with the nature of the patient's presentation and risk potential.

Finally, act on your findings, and continually reassess and evaluate your plan of care.

Scenario 3.1   Acute myocardial infarction

Mr Khan, a 48-year-old male of Asian origin, presents to the emergency department with a 30-minute history of non-radiating central chest pain and collapse.

He is able to talk. His respiratory rate is fast, regular and recorded as 26. There are no signs of central or peripheral cyanosis. His radial pulse is strong, regular and recorded as 70 bpm, this is in conjunction with a distal capillary nail bed refill time within two seconds. There is no evidence of external injuries from the collapse, although he has vomit down his shirt. He appears frightened, anxious and states his father died in his forties of a heart attack. He is pale, sweaty and clammy.

He works as a computer operator, has no previous medical history, smokes 20 low-tar cigarettes per day and is allergic to penicillin. He also appears to be grossly overweight.

D *Data* (scientific facts): Mr Khan is presenting with at least four prime risk factors for the development of CHD and an ischaemic episode. On arrival he has central chest pain, a history of vomiting and appears sweaty and clammy, all of which are symptoms of serious illness. In conjunction with the collapse, he will need one-to-one care within the resuscitation room, near to a defibrillator. AMI or the development of another life-threatening arrhythmia must be negated as soon as possible; the use of a cardiac monitor and the recording of a 12-lead ECG will achieve this.

Mr Khan is not portraying significant signs of physiological shock, but deterioration and sudden cardiac arrest are a real possibility.

E *Emotions* (intuition): Cardiac-related presentations are a high priority for all emergency clinicians; several national targets which are regularly audited need to be met to provide both quality and quantifiable evidence of clinical practice (DoH 2004).

The inexperienced clinician may not immediately recognize the seriousness of this presentation, although they should follow departmental policies. Senior clinicians will experientially know to follow the local policy for patients attending with chest pain.

A *Advantages*: Mr Khan's presenting history and clinical presentation should initiate a cascade of reactions from the clinician. The clinician must rule out a cardiac event or a dysrhythmia as the priority. Under national standards an ECG needs to be recorded within 15 minutes of arrival, with this presenting history it should be recorded immediately, and continual cardiac monitoring commenced. The advantage of administering anti-platelet agents and commencing high-flow oxygen as early as possible is vital to the patient's prognosis. His respiratory rate should be monitored in addition to the application of pulse oximetry to ascertain the patient's oxygenation status. A venous cannula should be inserted, most acute services will have a set protocol on which bloods are necessary at this stage; the clinician should use their professional judgement, as not all presentations are straightforward. Blood analysis should negate an electrolyte imbalance and a blood glucose will identify possible hyper/hypoglycaemia.

D *Disadvantages* (**differential diagnosis**): All patients presenting with chest pain are not necessarily having an AMI; they will, however, all need to be risk-assessed due to the potential seriousness of a missed infarction. Other common causes of chest pain are summarized in Table 3.4. There are several other life-threatening possibilities for Mr Khan's appearance, these include: acute aneurysm and pulmonary embolism, both of which will need to be negated.

EGG analysis using a systematic approach:

- Regular rhythm: each ventricular beat/QRS wave preceded by an atrial contraction or P wave.
- Constant P-R interval of 4 small squares.
- Normal QRS duration in leads I, aVR, V1–V4.

Table 3.4 Common causes of chest pain

Type of pain	Possible instigator
• Crushing – constricting	• Ischaemia
• Burning – dysphagia	• Oesophagitis
• Sharp – piercing – increases on inspiration and coughing	• Pleuritic – pericarditis – pneumonia
• Ripping – intrascapular chest to back	• Aortic dissection
• Pain on movement exercise	• Possible ischaemia
• Pain relieved by sitting forward	• Pericarditis
• Pain that increases when touched	• Musculoskeletal (trauma)
• Central chest pain at rest for > 30 seconds	• Possible AMI – Ischaemia

Note: Patients can use various terms to describe their pain. The expressions above are commonly used but no particular phrase guarantees a diagnosis. Look for other signs or clinical data that reinforce your suspicions.

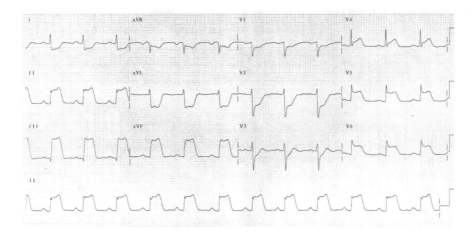

Figure 3.4   Inferior/lateral myocardial infarction

- Abnormal in leads II, III, aVF, V5 and V6, which demonstrate lengthening of the QRS complex involving the ST segment.
- Leads V1–V3 demonstrate ST segment depression.
- V5 and V6 demonstrate ST elevation.
- Leads II, III and aVF also have ST elevation.

Summary of findings

When analysing an ECG, it is vital that the inexperienced practitioner begins with a structured approach (identifying the origin of the conduction), otherwise there is the potential to overlook other vital data, heart block being a classic example.

This ECG demonstrates an acute infarction affecting both the lateral and inferior aspects of the heart. The ST depression in the anterior leads V1–V3 demonstrates evidence of reciprocal changes for the areas of infarction.

In combination with the presenting history, Mr Khan requires urgent treatment.

Treatment regimens for ACS

The Department of Health's document *Reforming Emergency Care* (DoH 2001), and National Service Framework for Coronary Heart Disease (2000) set specific targets for the administration of fibrinolytics or percutaneous coronary interventions (PCI) following the diagnosis of STEMI. These targets and their evidence base have recently been re-evaluated by the European Society for

Cardiology (ESC 2005). The findings reveal significant improvements can be made in patient morbidity and mortality rates if patients attending with either STEMI, or NSTEMI are treated as soon as possible with the use of percutaneous coronary interventions. Patients attending with clinical evidence of an ACS but no ST segment elevation need to be assessed for their potential risk of an acute thrombotic episode (ESC 2005).

Although patients attending with NSTEMI or ACS may demonstrate the same clinical findings as patients experiencing STEMI, they do not demonstrate the ECG changes associated with full thickness infarction and, therefore, do not meet the traditional criteria for immediate thrombolysis/PCI. Within clinical practice this can result in patients attending without the specifically targeted criteria receiving non-prioritized care despite the underpinning pathophysiological process and potential for full thickness infarction and sudden death. Patients presenting with chest pain and established left bundle branch block (LBBB) demonstrate a prime example.

The early identification of AMI and appropriate action, i.e., the administration of high-flow oxygen, nitrates, morphine, anti-emetics and anti-platelets in combination with possible thrombolytic therapy/percutaneous coronary interventions, can prevent and reduce the amount of damage the myocardium experiences, thereby limiting the future development of heart failure (ESC 2005).

Box 3.6 Summary of treatments

- **Anti-coagulants**: unfractionalized (UFH) and low molecular weight heparin (LMWH): true anti-coagulants prolonging clotting time reducing further clotting, enabling thrombus to disperse.
- **Anti-platelet agents**: aspirin and clopidogrel used together to reduce platelet aggregation in response to internal arterial damage (NICE 2004). Glycoprotein IIb/IIIa inhibitors are also used prior to PCI and in the treatment of NSTEMI; their use is currently under review by NICE.
- **Thrombolytics**: directly decompose the thrombus. Time-dependent reduction in morbidity and mortality rates.

Thrombolysis inclusion criteria:

- Presentation within 12 hours of the onset of chest pain in combination with ST-elevation of at least 2mm in two adjacent chest leads or 1mm in two adjacent limb leads. Evidence of posterior infarction and new bundle branch block are also included. Presentations between 12–14 hours may also be considered if signs and symptoms continue. Due to the associated risk of bleeding, thrombolytics also have a strict exclusion criteria.

- **Morphine/diamorphine**: reduce pain, anxiety and reduce preload, thereby removing potential strain on the heart.
- **Anti-emetics**: reduce nausea and vomiting thereby preventing further strain on the heart.
- **Glyceryl trinitrate (GTN)**: short-acting nitrate (vasodilators), which dilate coronary arteries, reduce myocardial oxygen demand and reduce both pre- and afterload.
- **Percutaneous coronary interventions**: direct dilation of the affected artery and use of stents to maintain artery patency.
- **Beta-blockers**: reduce heart rate and lower blood pressure, preventing further coronary events.
- **Statins**: reduce cholesterol levels in the blood and possibility of further events.

In patients presenting with UA or NSTEMI with a high risk for acute thrombotic complications (Box 3.4), early angiography with the possibility of percutaneous coronary intervention (PCI) has a clear benefit (Box 3.7).

Box 3.7 When patients benefit from immediate PCI

- In STEMI, PCI should be the treatment of choice (ECS 2005).
- Any contraindications to thrombolysis should signal immediate PCI.
- If the patient exhibits signs of cardiogenic shock, immediate PCI is indicated.
- PCI is indicated with late presentations, when major adverse cardiac events increase following thrombolysis.
- Within the first 3 hours of symptoms, both reperfusion strategies seem equally effective in reducing both the size and mortality rate associated with AMI.
- Between 3 and 12 hours PCI has a superior effect on myocardium preservation than thrombolysis.
- Primary PCI when compared to thrombolysis significantly reduced stroke development.

Therefore primary PCI is preferred over thrombolysis to reduce overall stroke development and to salvage myocardium (ESC 2005).

Scenario 3.2 Atrial fibrillation

Mrs Rhoads, a 78-year-old Caucasian female, presents with a vague history of dizziness, nausea and lethargy.

She states she hasn't felt right for a few weeks. Her respiratory rate is fast, regular and recorded as 23. There are signs of peripheral cyanosis. Her radial pulse is hard to locate, irregularly irregular and recorded as 127 bpm. This is in conjunction with a distal CRT exceeding 2 seconds, and the initial BP reads 110/68.

Mrs Rhoads appears pale and emaciated. She is orientated to time and place. Her pupils are equal and reactive to light.

Mrs Rhoads is a retired head schoolteacher, has no relevant previous medical history or allergies. She likes a glass of wine or sherry in the afternoon and becomes annoyed when questioned about her alcohol consumption.

D *Data* (scientific facts): Mrs Rhoads demonstrates an increased respiratory rate, evidence of cyanosis and poor perfusion, supported by the reduced CRT.

The blood pressure is within normal limits, although this is unusually low for someone of her age range not on anti-hypertensive medication, therefore this could indicate the beginning of haemodynamic collapse. The patient's pulse rate is tachycardic at 127; the irregularity of the pulse provides the experienced clinician with enough evidence to formulate a working diagnosis of atrial fibrillation (AF). The aetiology of atrial fibrillation is wide and therefore several potential instigators will need to be eliminated (Box 3.8).

E *Emotions* (intuition): a history of lethargy, dizziness and nausea in an elderly individual can signal many uncertainties to the clinician. The irregularity and rate of the pulse intuitively send the clinician down a cardiac pathway but drug toxicity, particularly Digoxin toxicity and electrolyte disturbances will need to be negated.

Box 3.8 Causes of atrial fibrillation
• Coronary heart disease
• Alcohol
• Hyperthyroidism
• Cardiomyopathy
• Infection (sepsis)
• AF can be idiopathic

To the inexperienced clinician Mrs Rhoads' presentation may not appear to be a classic cardiac-related emergency but, on the contrary, the underpinning cause is the most prevalent cardiac presentation in emergency care: that of atrial fibrillation.

In conjunction with the history of collapse, this patient will require further assessment within a high dependency area.

A *Advantages*: the application of supplementary oxygen and the regular monitoring of vital signs could curtail potential ischaemia development. The clinician must rule out a cardiac event or a dysrhythmia as the priority. With this presenting history the clinician will attach the patient to a cardiac monitor and record a 12-lead ECG.

Once the ECG or rhythm strip has been recorded, the clinician will move onto the United Kingdom Resuscitation Council's algorithm for tachycardias (Figure 3.6). A venous cannula and a request for blood analysis to rule out a cardiac event, electrolyte abnormality or metabolic disorder are essential. A blood glucose and urinalysis will be required and the patient's temperature should be monitored as hypo/hyperthermia can cause irregularity to the pulse rate.

Figure 3.5 demonstrates a narrow complex tachycardia. When a dysrhythmia is identified, there are two immediate questions the clinician needs to ask:

1   Is there a pulse or signs of circulation? If not, the advanced life support algorithm should be commenced.
2   Is the patient haemodynamically compromised or incapacitated?

In this case, Mrs Rhoads is physically stable although she may be exhibiting signs of compensatory shock development. Her ventricular rate varies between 70 and 140bpm and is irregularly irregular. The baseline or iso-electric line appears chaotic or unorganized and P waves cannot be clearly identified. There is no distinguishable P-R interval and therefore no relationship between the atria and the ventricles. The width of the QRS complex is less than three small squares; this rhythm therefore equates to a narrow complex, irregularly irregular tachycardia or fast atrial fibrillation.

D *Disadvantages* (**differential diagnosis**): Mrs Rhoads is pale, emaciated and has felt unwell for a while: this could indicate a more sinister pathology or an overactive thyroid gland. Box 3.8 highlighted the main causes of AF; these will need to be eliminated.

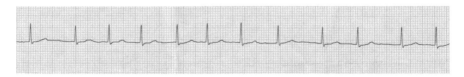

Figure 3.5   Atrial fibrillation

Atrial fibrillation

Prevalance and statistics

Atrial fibrillation is the most common cardiac arrhythmia, and is associated with an increased risk of embolus-related stroke, heart failure due to a reduced cardiac output and premature death (Bilal Iqbal et al. 2005). It affects approximately 4 per cent of over 65-year-olds in the US; this figure proliferates to 15 per cent by age 75 (Ezekowitz 1999). Majeed et al. (2001) suggest there are approximately 650,000 individuals diagnosed with AF in England and Wales. This is probably an underestimate as many people live with undiagnosed AF until a symptom manifests. Stewart et al. (2004) state that the prevalence of AF is increasing and that 1 in 100 of the UK population experience AF; this increases to 1 in 10 in the elderly. Most patients with AF require long-term pharmacological treatment, often including anti-coagulants; these medicines require constant monitoring which is expensive and time-consuming. The prevalence of AF-related hospitalizations has increased twofold to threefold over recent years (Stewart et al. 2004).

Pathophysiology

Individuals experiencing atrial fibrillation commonly present in one of three ways:

- First, and in the case of Mrs Rhoads, the history is of lethargy and a sensation of weakness, this is due to the slight reduction in cardiac output that the patient can experience.

- Second, failure of the heart as a pump; generally if heart disease is well established, the reduction in cardiac output would result in the patient presenting as haemodynamically compromised. Under normal circumstances coordinated atrial activity contributes to up to 20 per cent of the total cardiac output. In atrial fibrillation there is no coordinated atrial activity and the atria fail to contract resulting in the patient becoming compromised.

- Third, blood stagnates within the atria, resulting in clot formation; these clots are eventually fired around the circulation commonly resulting in a stroke (Chapter 10).

Treatments

Mrs Rhoads will be admitted for further comprehensive tests. Atrial fibrillation is a complex presentation to treat and its management is dependent on potential risk factors. NICE are currently reviewing AF guidelines which they aim to publish in 2006. The emergency management phase is covered within the RCUK tachycardia algorithm (Figure 3.6).

Cardioversion can re-establish a sinus rhythm although if the failure of the atria to pump effectively has led to stagnation of blood within the atria, the risk from embolism is high and the patient may need anticoagulation therapy prior to cardioversion. Medications are also available which pharmacologically cardiovert; these include amiodarone and flecainide.

If the AF is well established, the chances of cardioversion working are greatly reduced and drugs may be prescribed to reduce the ventricular response. Depending on the risk factors the patient may be prescribed long-term anticoagulant therapy.

 Scenario 3.3 Heart block

Mr Clarkson, a 63-year-old Caucasian male, presents after a close friend found him collapsed in his kitchen after experiencing a short period of dizziness. He denies having chest pain. His respiratory rate is regular and recorded as 32. There are no signs of central or peripheral cyanosis. His radial pulse is strong, regular and recorded as 27 bpm; this is in conjunction with a CRT exceeding 2 seconds. His blood pressure is 128/72. He appears pale and clammy, although orientated to time and place. Mr Clarkson states he had a heart attack five years ago. His only medication is the beta-blocker he takes each morning. He has no allergies.

D *Data* (scientific facts): from the primary data gathered while at rest Mr Clarkson exhibits poor peripheral perfusion and appears to be in a compensatory stage of shock; this manifests as a dramatic increase to his respiratory rate. In this case the pulse rate is not a good indicator of the development of shock. This is due to the beta-blockers he takes which may compromise the ability of his heart to compensate by speeding up via the fight or flight response. His radial pulse is regular although extremely slow.

E *Emotions* (intuition): the presenting history of dizziness and collapse could have several serious causes; the extreme bradycardia makes this a life-threatening emergency. The patient is therefore moved directly to the resuscitation room.

A *Advantages*: the RCUK bradycardia algorithm should be followed and supplementary oxygen commenced (Figure 3.7), if ischaemic changes are found on the ECG, anti-platelet medication should be given if no contraindications exist. Transdermal pacing pads must be quickly made available due to the potential for electrical failure of the heart's conduction system. Early specialist referral is essential as this patient will require pacing, in the meantime atropine and glucagon (the antidote to beta-blocker toxicity) should be made ready. An IV cannula will need to be sited and the early acquisition of bloods

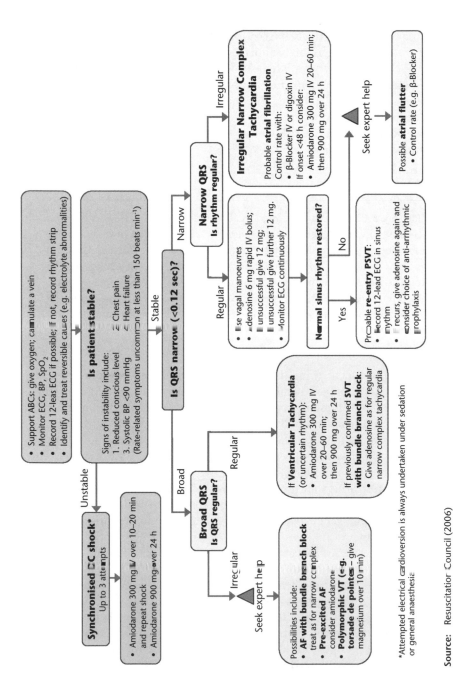

- Support ABCs; give oxygen; cannulate a vein
- Monitor ECG, BP, SpO₂
- Record 12-lead ECG if possible; if not, record rhythm strip
- Identify and treat reversible causes (e.g. electrolyte abnormalities)

Is patient stable?

Signs of instability include:
1. Reduced conscious level   2. Chest pain
3. Systolic BP <90 mmHg   4. Heart failure
(Rate-related symptoms uncommon at less than 150 beats min⁻¹)

Is QRS narrow (<0.12 sec)?

Unstable

Synchronised DC shock*
Up to 3 attempts

- Amiodarone 300 mg IV over 10–20 min and repeat shock
- Amiodarone 900 mg over 24 h

Stable

Broad

Broad QRS
Is QRS regular?

Regular

If Ventricular Tachycardia (or uncertain rhythm):
- Amiodarone 300 mg IV over 20–60 min; then 900 mg over 24 h

If previously confirmed SVT with bundle branch block:
- Give adenosine as for regular narrow complex tachycardia

Irregular

Seek expert help

Possibilities include:
- **AF with bundle branch block** treat as for narrow complex
- **Pre-excited AF** consider amiodarone
- **Polymorphic VT (e.g. torsade de pointes** – give magnesium over 10 min)

Narrow

Narrow QRS
Is rhythm regular?

Regular

- Use vagal manoeuvres
- Adenosine 6 mg rapid IV bolus; if unsuccessful give 12 mg; if unsuccessful give further 12 mg
- Monitor ECG continuously

Normal sinus rhythm restored?

Yes

Probable re-entry PSVT:
- Record 12-lead ECG in sinus rhythm
- If recurs, give adenosine again and consider choice of anti-arrhythmic prophylaxis

No

Seek expert help

Irregular

Irregular Narrow Complex Tachycardia
Probable **atrial fibrillation**
Control rate with:
- β-Blocker IV or digoxin IV
If onset <48 h consider:
- Amiodarone 300 mg IV 20–60 min; then 900 mg over 24 h

Possible **atrial flutter**
- Control rate (e.g. β-Blocker)

*Attempted electrical cardioversion is always undertaken under sedation or general anaesthesia

Source: Resuscitation Council (2006)

Figure 3.6 Tachycardia algorithm

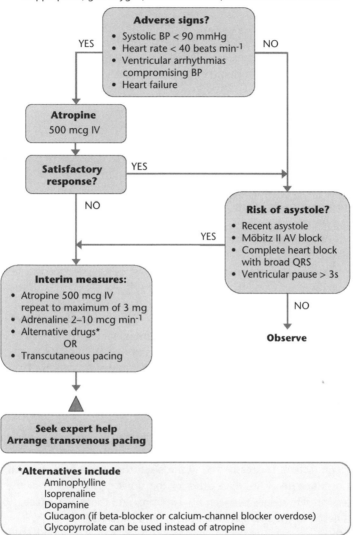

If appropriate, give oxygen, cannulate a vein, and record a 12-lead ECG

Adverse signs?
- Systolic BP < 90 mmHg
- Heart rate < 40 beats min⁻¹
- Ventricular arrhythmias compromising BP
- Heart failure

YES   NO

Atropine
500 mcg IV

Satisfactory response?   YES

NO

Risk of asystole?
- Recent asystole
- Möbitz II AV block
- Complete heart block with broad QRS
- Ventricular pause > 3s

YES

NO

Observe

Interim measures:
- Atropine 500 mcg IV repeat to maximum of 3 mg
- Adrenaline 2–10 mcg min⁻¹
- Alternative drugs*
  OR
- Transcutaneous pacing

**Seek expert help
Arrange transvenous pacing**

*Alternatives include
   Aminophylline
   Isoprenaline
   Dopamine
   Glucagon (if beta-blocker or calcium-channel blocker overdose)
   Glycopyrrolate can be used instead of atropine

Source: Resuscitation Council (2006) (Reproduced with permission)

Figure 3.7 Bradycardia algorithm

and their subsequent analysis are essential to the patient's prognosis as many blood abnormalities can result in severe episodes of bradycardia; these include hypothyroidism, and other metabolic disturbances.

D *Disadvantages* (differential diagnosis): other possible serious diagnoses that need to be negated include a stroke and acute myocardial infarction. Any presentation with a history of dizziness or collapse should include a blood glucose analysis.

Hypo/hyperthermia can cause irregularity to the pulse rate with hypothermia slowing the metabolic rate. If the patient is hypothermic, he should be warmed slowly as not to cause arrhythmias associated with sudden changes to core temperature (Houghton and Gray 2003).

Heart blocks pathophysiology

Over-vagal stimulation and beta-blocker toxicity can result in a profound bradycardia (Figure 3.8), paradoxically the patient may also demonstrate tachycardia. The working diagnosis is based on Mr Clarkson's extremely slow heart rate being insufficient to meet the demands of his body. This can be aggravated when extra strain is placed on the heart, resulting in the signs and symptoms of cardiogenic shock. The origin of the impulse can fail to produce a ventricular contraction resulting in syncope.

The heart rate of between 20 and 30bpm is suggestive of a ventricular escape rhythm, confirmed by the wide QRS complex. The origin of the instigating stimulus will be from a distal part of the conduction network or from the ventricles themselves (Box 3.9). There is a direct correlation between the origin of the impulse and its subsequent reliability. In other words electrical impulses that originate from the nodes are far more reliable than when they originate from ventricular cells where they are unpredictable and potentially lethal.

Box 3.9 The cardiac conducting system

Under normal physiology the Sinoatrial (SA) node is the heart's pacemaker, meaning an impulse from this collection of conducting fibres instigates myocardial contraction. The reason the SA node sets the pace is because it initiates a faster intrinsic rate of fire than either of the other cardiac nodes or the heart muscle. This rate ranges between 60–100bpm, and the rate is affected by the body's needs via the autonomic nervous system (Figure 3.8).

If there is a failure of the SA node to conduct an impulse to the atrioventricular (AV) node, the AV node will itself instigate the impulse and become the pacemaker with a rate between 40–60bpm. If this back-up mechanism also fails, impulses can be generated further down the conduction system. This includes the bundle of His and Purkinje fibres. These rates vary between 15–40bpm but are notoriously unreliable.

By understanding the rate/origin, the clinician can make an informed guess about the possible origin of heart blocks (although this provides a good rule of thumb, it is not always correct).

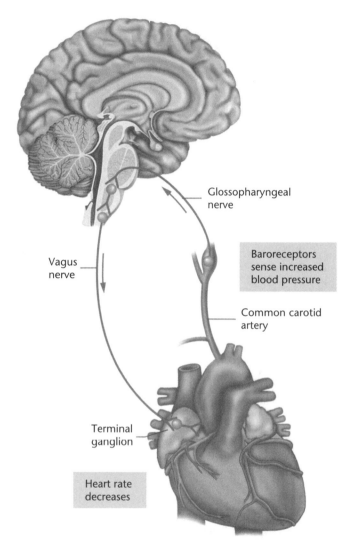

Glossopharyngeal
nerve

Baroreceptors
sense increased
blood pressure

Vagus
nerve

Common carotid
artery

Terminal
ganglion

Heart rate
decreases

Source: Saladin (2005)

Figure 3.8 An autonomic reflex arc in the regulation of blood pressure

Degrees of heart block

Type one: first degree (Figure 3.9)

An increased interval between atrial activity and the commencement of ventricular activity (prolongation of the P-R interval). This prolongation can

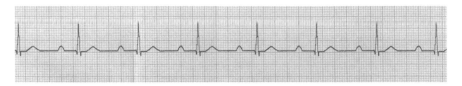

Figure 3.9 First degree heart block

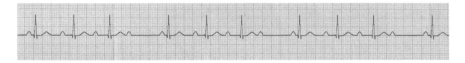

Figure 3.10 Second degree heart block type I

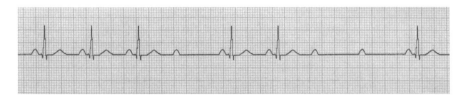

Figure 3.11 Second degree heart block type II

be a normal variant and asymptomatic although drug therapy, hypokalaemia and ischaemic heart disease have all been identified as attributing factors.

Type two: second degree

There are three categories:

1. *Mobitz type I or Wenckebach* (Figure 3.10): Increasing delay in AV conduction with each successive complex until ultimately failure of conduction occurs. The sight of the block is usually high in the junctional tissues, near or within the AV node and can simply arise from periods of high vagal activity (during sleep). The Wenckebach phenomenon is regarded as a relatively stable form of heart block and a pacemaker is not required unless the dropped beats result in the individual becoming haemodynamically compromised.
2. *Mobitz type II* (Figure 3.11): Most P waves are conducted. The P-R interval is generally constant. Occasionally an atrial contraction (P wave) fails to produce a ventricular contraction (QRS complex). Results from abnormal conduction below the AV node (bundle of His) and can progress without warning to complete heart block.

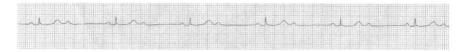

Figure 3.12 Second degree heart block (2:1)

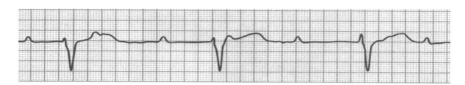

Figure 3.13 Complete heart block

3. *Second degree heart block (2:1)* (Figure 3.12): Alternate P waves are not followed by a QRS complex (not conducted). The 2:1 AV block stands alone because it is impossible to deduce if the non-conducted P waves would have been the same as, or longer than, the conducted P waves.

Type three: complete heart block (Figure 3.13)

Complete disruption of the conduction sequence, resulting in the atria and ventricles working independently with the ventricles being governed by an escape rhythm. A combination of bradycardia and wide ventricular complexes should alert the practitioner. Temporary pacing is indicated regardless of the individual's haemodynamic state.

Scenario 3.4 Ventricular tachycardia

Ms Veronica Deville, a 24-year-old Caucasian female, well known to the department, presents complaining of a severe headache, chest pain and shortness of breath.

She is sweating profusely, appears pale and is hyperventilating. She is very anxious and when questioned admits snorting several lines of cocaine over the last 8 hours in combination with several glasses of wine.

Her respiratory rate is fast, regular and recorded as 34. There are no signs of central or peripheral cyanosis. Her radial pulse is bounding, regular and recorded as 140 bpm; this is in conjunction with a distal CRT within two seconds. Her blood pressure is recorded as 158/106. Ms Deville is orientated to time and place.

She has had several previous attendances due to alcohol intoxication and cocaine use.

She smokes 40 low-tar cigarettes per day and has no known allergies.

D *Data* (scientific facts): Ms Deville's presenting history identifies several high risk factors these include: tachypnoea, hypertension, tachycardia and in combination with the physical appearance signal a severe increase in the sympathetic response.

This response can be instigated by drugs that increase the sympathetic response (sympathomimetics), i.e., amphetamines (speed) and cocaine. These powerful and commonly abused recreational drugs can lead to major episodes of arterial spasm, inducing ischaemia to major organs such as the brain or heart and extreme episodes of hypertension. They can also initiate extremely fast tachycardias, which, in this case is confirmed by the pulse.

E *Emotions* (intuition): the experienced clinician would intuitively recognize the seriousness of this presentation. The patient's physical presentation includes a sweaty, pale appearance. Clinically, the seriousness of this finding is consolidated by the erratic respiratory and pulse rates. In most cardiac pathology a failing heart will result in hypotension, but because of the action of the stimulants taken, the arterioles have been constricted resulting in a dramatically increased afterload and blood pressure.

The experienced clinician will immediately admit the patient to the resuscitation room and commence high flow supplementary oxygen, while attaching the patient to a cardiac monitor.

This presentation is life-threatening and the possibility of the patient experiencing a cardiac arrhythmia a real threat. The immediate conductional rhythm will be established via a rhythm strip, a full view of the electrical activity of the heart will also be required so a 12-lead ECG will be recorded to negate an AMI.

A *Advantages*: reassurance and a calm atmosphere are conducive to helping the patient relax and induce a reduction to the sympathetic response. The quick application of oxygen is paramount as this may prevent an ischaemic episode or respiratory failure as the patient will not be able to maintain a respiratory rate of this proportion for a prolonged period; pulse oximetry should be monitored and an arterial blood gas may be taken to ascertain respiratory function. A cannula will need to be inserted and bloods taken, depending on local policy, a troponin level could be recorded. An anxiolytic such as diazepam could be given in conjunction with a small-titrated dose of morphine and an anti-emetic. If the ECG reveals ST segment elevation, the on-call cardiologist's opinion should be sought as many departments have a specific treatment protocol for possible stimulant-induced ST elevation.

A *Disadvantages* (differential diagnosis): AMI and narrow or broad complex tachycardias are the prime causes of concern. A sinus tachycardia is also a possibility due to effects of the stimulants.

Further data should include identifying risk factors for AMI, blood glucose examination, regular neurological and temperature monitoring, as stimulants can cause hyperpyrexia.

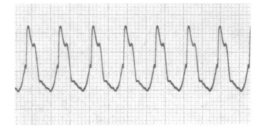

Figure 3.14   Broad complex tachycardia (VT)

Some clinicians advocate the early administration of anxiolytics or beta-blockers to relieve some of the effects of stimulants. Although Ms Deville demonstrates a dangerously high respiratory rate, this may be due to hyperventilation rather than hypoxia and in combination with the blood pressure she is not haemodynamically compromised.

Figure 3.14 demonstrates a regular broad complex tachycardia with a rate around 180; this is identified as an unstable ventricular tachycardia due to the abnormal width of the QRS complexes (refer to stage 5 of the ECG guide). As with all cardiac arrhythmias, the clinician will use the ECG data to reinforce their physical findings. The RCUK guidelines for tachycardias (Figure 3.6) will be used to guide the subsequent treatment plan. This easy-to-follow algorithm provides the practitioner with a clear pathway of treatment dependent on the patient's clinical condition. In the case of Ms Deville, there are minimal signs of compromise, therefore following the algorithm, the anti-arrhythmic amiodarone will be administered with close cardiac monitoring as arrhythmias may development.

Cardiac arrest synopsis

Cardiac arrest can be defined as the sudden or acute cessation of the heartbeat and subsequently cardiac function, resulting in the loss of effective circulation and therefore, incompatible with life.

The RCUK have recently updated their guidelines on advanced life support (RCUK 2006). These guidelines provide a structured protocol-based approach to the emergency management of patients experiencing cardiac arrest (Figure 3.15).

Most cardiac arrests within the hospital environment are predictable events, with many early warning signs and symptoms (RCUK 2006).

The ALS guidelines are initially based on the chain of survival outlined in Table 3.5.

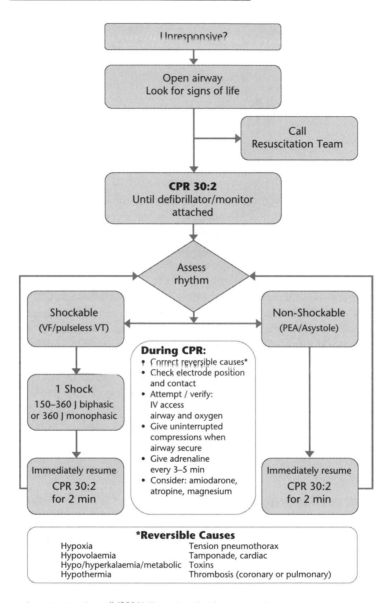

Source. Resuscitation Council (2006) (Reproduced with permission)

Figure 3.15 Adult advanced life support algorithm

Chapter 2 identified many of the early warning signs synonymous with cardiac arrest; the following section describes the arrest rhythms and the associated ECG changes. The reader is referred to the RCUK guidelines for in-depth guidance.

Table 3.5 The chain of survival

Act	Rationale
• Early recognition of associated signs and call for help • Early cardiopulmonary resuscitation (CPR) • Early defibrillation • Post-resuscitation care	• Prevention is better than cure • Cerebral oxygenation while buying time • To restart organized electrical activity and cardiac output • To maintain adequate circulation • Prevent further arrests • To restore quality of life

All clinicians working within emergency care need to be familiar with the cardiac rhythms synonymous with cardiac arrest and the two pathways of management (Figure 3.15).

Advanced life support

The treatment of cardiac arrest centres on achieving cerebral and vital organ perfusion until definitive treatment such as defibrillation can be delivered or an instigating cause identified and treated.

Shockable rhythms

This requires a cardiac monitor to identify an underlying rhythm. If the rhythm is pulseless ventricular tachycardia (PVT) or ventricular fibrillation (VF), the application of an electrical current or defibrillation to the heart muscle may result in the chaotic rhythm and fibrillating muscle mass becoming organized again, and the patient regaining a cardiac output/pulse. VF and PVT are commonly associated with AMI and have the lowest mortality rate when early treatment is initiated. Therefore if the cause of the cardiac arrest is due to electrical faults such as ventricular fibrillation, defibrillation is the key to management (Figure 3.15).

Non-shockable rhythms

Two other rhythms are associated with the arrested patient: the first is asystole, which means without output, i.e., an absence of electromechanical activity throughout the heart. This, therefore, cannot be defibrillated and the management centres on basic life support. Traditionally referred to as a 'flat line' and hence the need to check lead attachments are correct. This arrhythmia has the highest mortality rate, causes include over-vagal stimulation.

The second is pulseless electrical activity (PEA). PEA can be defined as an organized electrical rhythm without a cardiac output/pulse, i.e., the patient is pulseless despite a potentially normal electrical rhythm. Common causes include hypovolaemia and hypoxia, in PEA the cause for the arrest should be established and addressed in order to restore a spontaneous circulation. Box 3.10 lists the reversible causes of cardiac arrest.

Box 3.10   Reversible causes of cardiac arrest (Four Hs and 4 Ts)

- **H**ypovolaemia
- **H**ypothermia
- **H**ypoxia
- **H**ypo/Hyper kalaemia (electrolye imbalance)
- **T**ension Pneumothorax
- **T**amponard – Cardiac
- **T**hromboembolic
- **T**oxic

Both are managed on the non-shockable side of the algorithm with the identification of an underlying alteration to normal physiology paramount to treatment success (Figure 3.15).

Conclusion

Cardiac emergencies offer the clinician an excellent opportunity to really make a difference to the patients in their care. Good clinical practice directly reflects on patient morbidity and mortality rates. The philosophy that prevention is better than cure is also relevant as the quick thinking and dynamic practitioner can recognize serious pathology at an early stage and by instigating treatment prevent the patient from clinical or physical deterioration.

4   Minor injury and illness

Claire Washbourne

Introduction

In recent years emergency care has undergone dramatic changes, particularly in the delivery of minor injury and illness care. This work stream accounts for approximately 50 per cent of emergency presentations (DoH 2006). The aim of this chapter is to provide practitioners new to the speciality, with a structured approach for undertaking an initial assessment of patients who present with a minor injury or illness. Pertinent issues and potential pitfalls are highlighted with the intention of guiding the reader through the process of history taking and examination.

Diagnosis, management and treatment of the most frequently seen presentations, including differential diagnosis, will be presented in order to raise awareness of potential pitfalls (red flag warnings).

History taking

The importance of accurate history taking and documentation cannot be over-emphasized. The questioning pattern suggested here is widely used when assessing patients with minor injuries or illness and should enable the assessor to decide on the priorities of care for each individual patient.

When

- Has the event just occurred or has time elapsed for other symptoms to occur?
- Is the presentation delayed, if so, why?

How

- Acting out the mechanism of injury to establish the injury is quick and clarifies details that are often 'lost' in translation.
- On occasion the patient is uncertain of the mechanism of injury, this should be documented; a loss of consciousness preceding or since the event should be excluded to ensure this was not a contributing factor.
- When the history of the injury does not necessarily relate to the presenting signs and symptoms, it may not be appropriate to question further at initial assessment, concerns should be relayed to colleagues in order that help or referral to other agencies can be offered, e.g. non-accidental injury, alcohol/drug abuse.

Why

- 'Why' links closely to 'how' used as a trigger to raise the 'bigger picture' questions of has this happened before or could this occurrence have been prevented?
- A presentation, no matter how minor, can be an early symptom of a much larger problem. As health professionals we have a responsibility to evaluate the significance of the presentation and address immediate issues or alert the appropriate agencies for follow-up.
- Does this patient keep presenting? Are we missing something?

Who

- Who is affected by this situation? Has this event affected their ability to care for themselves or others?
- Is the patient's occupation going to be affected by this event? Are they able to work? Were unsafe practices occurring and should the patient inform their employer for health and safety at work reasons?

Where

- Knowledge of where events occurred draws an accurate picture, highlighting clinical risks e.g. exposure to infections such as tetanus.
- Practitioners should be aware of conditions commonly not seen in the UK, e.g., Myiasis – a condition caused by larvae from flies burrowing under the skin, occurring in parts of Africa.

What

- The object that caused the injury can assist in determining the structures that are most likely to be damaged. A sharp penetrating injury with a knife is likely to cut through tendons or nerves, while crush injuries cause soft tissue swelling that compresses nerves, producing a temporary reduction in sensation (neuropraxia) that resolves as the swelling reduces.

Minor injuries: wrist and hand

History

A natural reflex action during a fall is for the victim to put their hand out to break the fall and prevent injury. The abbreviation FOOSH is often used to minimize documentation time and stands for fall on outstretched hand. In the elderly reaction times may be reduced, so clarity must be established regarding mechanism of injury and whether, on making contact with the ground, body weight was transferred through an extended or flexed hand.

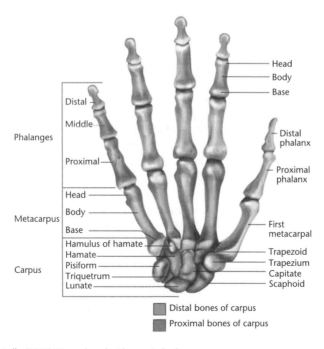

Source: Saladin (2005) (Reproduced with permission)

Figure 4.1   The right wrist and hand

Carrying shopping or a cyclist applying the brakes could produce a flexed hand being involved with the mechanism of injury. The patient may report that the event happened so quickly that they cannot recall what position their hand was in, but clues to the event can be seen in abrasions on the palm implying FOOSH, with wounds to the dorsum of the hand or 'knuckles' suggestive of a type of flexed wrist injury. A condition that commonly presents following a FOOSH is that of a scaphoid fracture, where the patient will often say that they had vague pain in their wrist at the time of injury, but ignored it because they had full movement and so presumed that no bones were broken. Some hours later an increasing pain develops, leading to swelling and a dramatic reduction in normal wrist and thumb movements.

Before any conclusions are drawn, it is important to exclude any other more significant symptoms that may have contributed to the fall such as a cardiac or neurological event. Recollection of events prior to, during and after the fall is important and any 'gap' in memory may suggest a loss of consciousness indicating further observation and investigation to exclude a more serious condition. Head, neck and facial injuries should be excluded if the mechanism of injury produced a sudden jolting force.

Punching type injuries often associated with assaults, usually result in injury to the dorsum of the hand. A detailed history will be necessary if a wound is present. If the patient has punched someone in the mouth, there is an increased potential for infection from a human bite and the presence of a foreign body, such as a tooth, needs to be excluded by X-ray of the soft tissues. The patient may be unwilling to disclose the full history due to feelings of guilt or liability, but frankness should be encouraged in order for appropriate treatment to occur.

Rotational injuries to the fingers can occur during an assault when the fingers are restrained, or in situations when fingers are removed quickly from a crush mechanism of injury, e.g., shut in car door.

Sporting injuries, usually involving sudden contact with the ball at close range as in basketball, netball, cricket, football and rugby, can cause hyperextension, flexion, abduction or adduction injuries to the fingers.

Repetitive movements, in particular to the wrist, can produce pain in the wrist and forearm, often the result of flexing or gripping the fingers for long periods of time or performing repeated movements of the wrist that are out with the usual pattern of a person's normal activity.

Minor burns to the hand are usually sustained in domestic accidents in the home during cooking. Be wary of those caused by electrical appliances as an electric shock can disrupt the electrical sequence of the heart and produce a full thickness injury that is not initially evident.

Examination findings/anatomy

Look

The most significant finding is deformity, which may be seen in the 'dinner fork' appearance of a displaced fractured distal radius (Figure 4.2). Finger joint swelling particularly around the proximal interphalangeal joint (PIPJ) is suggestive of joint disruption and/or injury to the collateral ligaments.

Deformity presents in the fingers following dislocation of ligaments and extensor tendon rupture at the distal interphalangeal joint (DIPJ) in which the distal phalanx appears to 'droop' out of alignment with the rest of the digit.

Bruising can be indicative of a significant soft tissue injury, particularly around joints. Bruising on the palmar/volar aspect may suggest a fracture or injury to the volar plate, located over the PIPJ.

A bruised appearance under a fingernail is usually produced following a crush injury when the nail is squashed against or lifted from the nail bed. Being a very vascular area, bleeding occurs, and because the blood is contained in a confined area, it collects, forming what is known as a subungal haematoma. In some cases the developing haematoma places so much pressure on the nerve endings of the finger that the patient may present some hours later in great distress due to the pain. That pain is only eased once the haematoma is released by making a hole in the nail, a procedure called trephining.

Feel

For the inexperienced practitioner differentiating between soft tissue and bony tenderness can be problematic. Asking the patient to point to where the

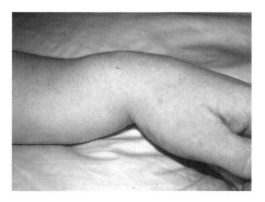

Note: This is typical of a Colles fracture but could also be the result of a fracture of the distal radius and ulna bones

Source: Reproduced with permission of the Royal College of Surgeons.
Available at: www.edu.rcsed.ac.uk

Figure 4.2 Dinner fork deformity

focus of pain is located should be established, initially avoid this area. Work from the joint above the injury, moving systematically down along the entire length of each bone by gently squeezing the individual bones between the index finger and thumb, finishing at the area of focused pain. An area of 'point' tenderness will usually relate to bony tenderness, as the patient may sharply withdraw the limb in response to the pain and it is reasonable to suspect a fracture may be present. The pain produced with soft tissue tenderness tends to manifest itself over a wider area.

Familiarizing yourself with the anatomical position of the bones in relation to surface anatomy comes with practice and exposure to the common presentations. From a medico-legal standpoint identifying the location of the scaphoid bone should be a priority in your learning because failure to recognize possible injury to this bone could have long-term detrimental consequences for the patient if overlooked. Any tenderness in the anatomical snuffbox, or volar aspect of the wrist over the scaphoid bone, is suggestive of a fracture and the significance of that finding should be conveyed to the patient at the time.

The minimum standard for assessing sensation to the fingers should involve touching each finger in turn and a comparison made with the other limb. The patient may have total numbness but more often they will describe a sensation of the digit feeling 'different' or 'sleepy', which is significant of nerve injury or may be neuropraxia.

Move

For the purpose of initial assessment the minimum standard of assessment should include the basic movements of flexion, extension, rotation, ulna and radial deviation with any reduction to normal range documented.

Flexing and extending the fingers should reveal any rotational deformity or reduced ROM suggestive of fracture or tendon rupture.

The ability to rotate the thumb at the metacarpal phalangeal joint (MCPJ) provides sufficient evidence to exclude significant loss of normal function.

Initial intervention

Pain assessment and the administration of analgesia are helpful for the patient and assist with physical examination at a later stage. Elevation of the hand or wrist in a sling in the immediate hours after injury greatly reduces the development of soft tissue swelling that often inhibits movement and produces pain.

Cryotherapy (ice packs) should be used with caution by avoiding application directly to fingers, as this could complicate determining sensory perception at a later stage.

Applying direct firm pressure in conjunction with elevation of the affected area should control active bleeding; medical attention should be sought if the flow cannot be stemmed after applying simple measures of pressure and elevation. If there is any suspicion of fracture, nerve or tendon damage it is pertinent to advise the patient to remain fasted so that emergency surgery is not delayed. Any jewellery on the affected limb should be removed.

> **Scenario 4.1**   Minor injuries: wrist and hand
>
> A 70-year-old lady is brought to the emergency department by ambulance following a fall in the street; she is able to walk into the department. On arrival she is alert and orientated but appears clammy and complains of pain in her right wrist, with reduced range of movement. An obvious deformity is visible over the distal radius/ulna area of her arm although there is no open wound.

D *Data* (scientific facts): initial data should exclude any history of loss of consciousness, chest pain or head injury prior to the event that may have contributed to the fall. Mechanism of injury should be established i.e. tripping on the pavement and landing on an outstretched hand. Baseline observation will be recorded and an assessment of circulation, sensation and movement. A wrist X-ray will be requested which shows an impacted fractured distal radius.

E *Emotions* (intuition): focusing immediately on a deformity can detract attention from a significant instigator to the injury, i.e., collapse or head injury. The patient may live alone or be the main carer for a spouse, and an injury that reduces a patient's independence may be a cause for concern. The patient's social situation should always be included in the initial assessment in order that prompt, appropriate discharge can be expedited.

A *Advantages*: pain assessment should be undertaken and pain relief administered to enable a thorough secondary examination. The wrist should be immobilized, to prevent further injury and to assist with pain relief, and elevated in a sling to reduce the amount of swelling around the fracture site. Jewellery should be removed from the fingers and wrist of the affected hand as they can restrict blood flow as the soft tissues swell during the inflammatory process.

D *Disadvantages* (differential diagnoses): the assessor should establish other injuries, such as head or shoulder injuries, which may have led to injury of the cervical spine. Haematomas and fractures can cause nerve damage and disruption to circulation; therefore, frequent reassessment is required in the initial phase of the presentation.

Injuries to the elbow and the scaphoid bone should also be excluded.

Minor injuries: treatment and management

Table 4.1 provides a guide to the expected treatment and management of the most common minor injuries. The list is not exhaustive and local variations in

Table 4.1 Management and treatment of common minor injuries

Injury	Management	Treatment
Colles fracture (Figure 4.3) Fractured distal radius with dorsal displacement	Pain relief Haematoma block Manipulation Application POP Fracture clinic follow-up	Application of below-elbow plaster of Paris (POP) back slab and sling
Smiths fracture Fractured distal radius with volar displacement	Pain relief Haematoma block Manipulation Application POP Referral to orthopaedic team for internal fixation under general anaesthetic	Application of above-elbow full POP High elevation prior to surgery to minimize soft tissue swelling
Confirmed scaphoid fracture (Figure 4.4)	Pain relief Follow up next fracture clinic	Application of scaphoid cast High arm sling
Anatomical snuffbox tenderness No fracture seen on X-ray	Treated as possible scaphoid fracture Pain relief Follow up fracture clinic 7–10 days time	Application of scaphoid cast or wrist splint with thumb extension (refer to local policy) High arm sling
Undisplaced fracture of distal end metacarpal	Neighbour strapping or volar slab POP depending on patient's pain Follow up in next fracture or hand clinic	Application neighbour strapping or volar slab POP
Displaced or angulated fracture of distal end or shaft metacarpal (Figure 4.5)	Possible manipulation under local anaesthetic Discuss management with on call plastics or orthopaedics depending on local policy Follow up in next fracture or hand clinic or possible admission for internal fixation	Application volar slab POP or Zimmer splint

Injury	Management	Treatment
Undisplaced fractured distal phalanx (finger)	Protective mallet or Zimmer splint	Application of mallet or Zimmer splint High sling initially
Subungal haematoma	Exclude fracture of underlying bone with an X-ray Release haematoma by trephining	Trephine Finger dressing High sling initially
Rupture of extensor tendon to distal phalanx of finger 'Mallet deformity' +/− avulsion fracture	X-ray to exclude avulsion fracture Mallet splint or 'Mexican hat' Zimmer splint Follow up orthopaedic or hand therapy clinic	Application Mallet splint or 'Mexican hat' Zimmer splint
Rupture of Ulna collateral ligament Thumb	If no laxity of MCPJ, follow up in orthopaedic or hand clinic If laxity, seek advice from orthopaedic or hand specialist	Thumb spica Temporary Zimmer splinting prior to possible surgical repair

practice may exist, its purpose is to highlight the many skills required by an emergency practitioner to care for this patient group.

Red flags

Anatomical snuffbox (ASB) tenderness is suggestive of a fracture to the scaphoid bone if trauma has occurred. Subtle symptoms such as pain on gripping when using their thumb or leaning bodyweight through their hand should not be dismissed, particularly if there is delay in the patient presenting.

Rotational deformity of the fingers noted when asking the patient to flex their fingers is indicative of a fracture to a metacarpal.

Inability to extend the distal phalanx of a finger is suggestive of a rupture of the extensor tendon.

Although rare, Lunate dislocation presents with a history of trauma, swelling and tenderness over the dorsum of the affected hand.

Patients presenting with soft tissue tenderness and swelling over the distal radius and forearm, with no significant history of trauma, should not be X-rayed initially. The condition may be tendonitis, which is often caused by

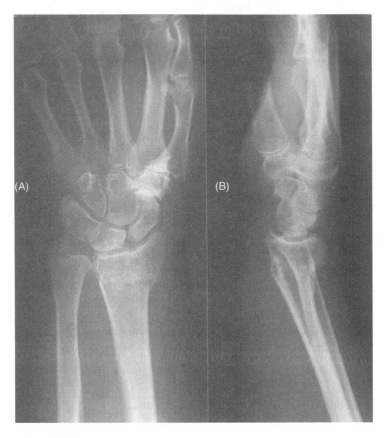

Source: Begg (2005)

Figure 4.3 (A) PA and (B) lateral view showing a Colles fracture with a typical dinner fork deformity

repetitive movements, a crepitus sensation can be palpated over the extensor tendons and X-ray examination would be unnecessary.

The elbow

History

Due to its anatomical position the elbow is most vulnerable to injury following a fall, when the mechanism of injury is rapid and the patient tries to prevent injury to the face by landing on outstretched hands, e.g., a cyclist who brakes sharply and propels over the handlebars. On landing, the direct force of the patient's bodyweight is transferred onto the hands through the wrist to the forearm, often leading to a fracture of the head/proximal end of the radius.

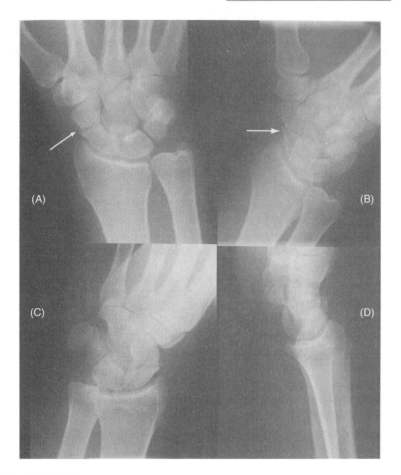

Source: Begg (2005)

Figure 4.4 Scaphoid series with a fracture through the waist of the scaphoid (arrow): (A) PA (B) PA (C) AP oblique (D) lateral

Initially significant injury may not be apparent, because normal function is maintained, but over a period of hours swelling develops in the joint space due to bleeding from the fracture, movements of extension and rotation reduce and produce pain.

Falls can result in direct trauma to the elbow, producing fractures of the olecranon, which has implications for the ligaments and tendons that attach to that bone.

Dislocation in an adult would be rare but is a common presentation in paediatrics sustained by toddlers when they are lifted up by one arm leading to a 'pulled elbow'.

Repetitive movements of the elbow, particularly in combination with

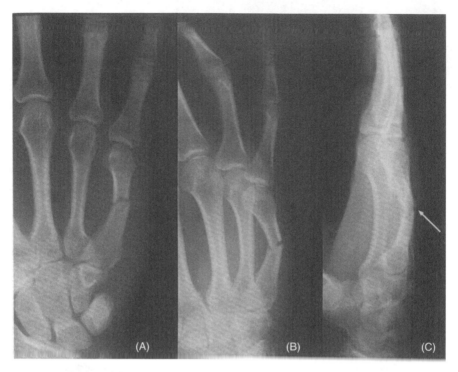

Note: The degree of forward angulation is optimally demonstrated on the lateral, and completely unappreciated on the PA

Source: Begg (2005)

Figure 4.5 (A) PA (B) oblique and (C) lateral views showing a fracture of the shaft of the 5th metacarpal

prolonged gripping of fingers, can lead to inflammation of the tendon that inserts into the radial head leading to a condition called epicondylitis or 'tennis elbow' or 'golfer's elbow'.

The olecranon bursa can become inflamed due to prolonged pressure; infection can occur as a result of very minor trauma, like an abrasion.

Examination findings/relevant anatomy

Look

Deformity is not obvious, if a dislocation has occurred it would be more apparent when the arm is held in fixed extension. Likewise significant swelling and bruising around this joint are more likely to be seen when the olecranon has been fractured or displaced.

Anterior

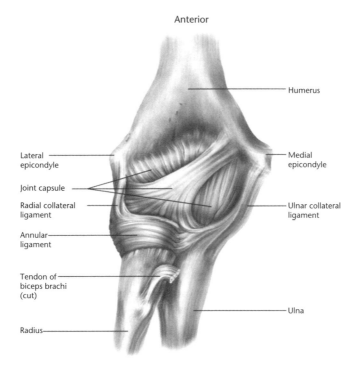

Humerus

Lateral epicondyle

Medial epicondyle

Joint capsule

Radial collateral ligament

Ulnar collateral ligament

Annular ligament

Tendon of biceps brachi (cut)

Ulna

Radius

Source: Saladin (2005) (Reproduced with permission)

Figure 4.6 The elbow joint anterior view

Feel

The following bony prominences should be palpated to exclude fracture:

- Medial epicondyle
- Lateral epicondyle
- Olecranon
- Radial head.

Distal sensation and circulation should be assessed by comparing sensation in all digits in that hand with the opposite side, along with capillary refill time, which should not exceed two seconds.

Move

Movements of flexion and extension should be assessed; rotation of the wrist is a valuable way of evaluating whether a fracture of the radial head should be considered, this movement causes rotation as it articulates with the capitellum.

Initial intervention

In the acute phase the patient appears in obvious discomfort; pain assessment and the administration of analgesia should be the priority along with the cleaning of any open wounds, which is common with this presentation of a fall.

Ice packs may be of benefit, as immobilization of the limb in a sling may prove problematic due to the patient being unwilling to move their elbow to 90 degrees due to pain causing tension in the muscles of the shoulder, and upper and lower arm. Benefit can be gained from supporting the weight of the arm allowing the muscles to relax, this should not be forced, especially if the patient will shortly have an X-ray and ideally their pain will have been relieved before the X-ray is performed.

Red flags

Joint sepsis should be suspected in a hot, swollen and inflamed elbow and would require immediate referral.

Any loss of sensation or delayed capillary refill should be brought to the attention of senior staff for further examination.

Table 4.2 Management and treatment of elbow injuries

Diagnosis	Management	Treatment
Undisplaced fracture radial head	Referral to fracture clinic Analgesia	Sling/collar and cuff
Displaced fractured olecranon	Referral to orthopaedic team for internal fixation	Above-elbow POP prior to surgery Elevation in sling/collar and cuff
Dislocation	Manipulation	Distraction tactics at the time of manipulation
Epicondylitis	Refrain from the activity causing the pain Simple pain relief such as Paracetamol and/or NSAIDs Steroid injection by GP or orthopaedic specialist if pain is prolonged	
Olecranon Bursitis	Exclude infection Rest Short course of NSAIDs	

The shoulder

History

Due to its structure the shoulder joint can be vulnerable to injury, with common histories ranging from landing directly on the anterior aspect of the joint, direct upward pressure into the joint when landing on an outstretched hand or elbow, or external rotation when the arm is thrust in a posterior direction. The close proximity of the head, neck and clavicle means that injury to those areas should be excluded from the outset and appropriate action taken if identified, e.g., neck immobilization or commencing neurological observations.

Close questioning of what predisposed the injury or fall should be undertaken to exclude neurological or cardiac events that may have led to a loss of consciousness or balance, particularly in the elderly who may delay their presentation (e.g., humeral fractures).

Dislocations present with sudden, severe pain and loss of function isolated to the shoulder, with the patient often preferring to stand in order to adopt a leaning forward stance to allow the arm to hang, using the counter-traction of gravity in an attempt to relieve pressure on the joint. Obvious deformity can be masked by clothing, so clarification of dislocation may require moving the patient to an area where there is space to assist the patient

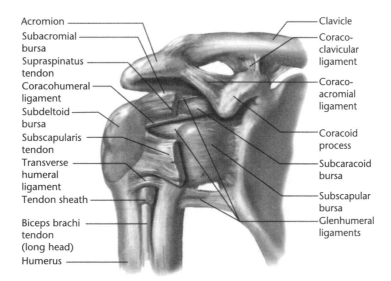

Source: Saladin (2005) (Reproduced with permission)

Figure 4.7   The shoulder (humoroscapular) joint

to undress and allow a more thorough assessment. If a dislocation is suspected, Entonox can be used while awaiting intravenous (IV) access, medical attention, and immediate titration of IV analgesia prior to sending the patient for a shoulder X-ray.

Direct blunt trauma to the posterior aspect of the shoulder is unlikely to produce more than soft tissue inflammation to the muscles of the rotator cuff. A significant force, such as falling from a height or a motor cyclist at speed landing on the posterior aspect of their shoulder, could produce a fracture of the scapula. However, the scapula is a robust bone and if a fracture has occurred, other injuries should be considered such as lung contusions, fractures of the ribs or spine.

Examination findings/relevant anatomy

Look
Deformity will often only be apparent once the chest and shoulder area are exposed and compared to the opposite side. Encouraging the patient to support the weight of their affected side while flexed, with their other hand and asking the patient to relax their neck and shoulder muscles can produce a more diagnostic view.

Swelling is not always apparent due to the large muscle bulk of the rotator cuff, localized swelling over the acromioclavicular joint (ACJ) is indicative of ligament and tendon disruption.

Bruising can be an indication of either dislocation, soft tissue injury or fracture at that site, a 'pooling' effect of bruising around the elbow, due to gravity, may be associated with a fracture of the shaft of the proximal end of the humerus.

Feel
Identifying specific points of bony tenderness over the proximal humerus can be problematic due to extensive covering of the muscles groups that make up the rotator cuff. Palpating the bony prominences of the clavicle and ACJ can quickly identify areas of injury.

Comparing sensation over the lateral aspect of the bicep area and identifying a deficit can be indicative of an axillary nerve lesion and must be assessed, particularly before and after manipulation of a shoulder dislocation

Move
Accurate assessment can be hindered by a patient in pain, but must include flexion, extension, abduction, adduction, and internal and external rotation.

Initial intervention

- Viewing the shoulder
- Identifying/negating dislocation
- Pain assessment
- Assessing movement
- Immobilization in broad arm sling.

Table 4.3 Management and treatment of shoulder injuries

Diagnosis	Management	Treatment
Dislocation	Relocation under sedation Check X-ray to confirm repositioning Fracture clinic follow-up	Assist with monitoring patient's vital signs during manipulation Application of collar and cuff sling or poly-sling once relocation achieved
Subluxation	Follow up fracture clinic	Sling/collar and cuff
ACJ sprain ACJ rupture	Referral for physiotherapy Pain relief Follow up fracture clinic Pain relief	Sling/collar and cuff Sling/collar and cuff
Fracture clavicle	Follow up fracture clinic Pain relief	Sling/collar and cuff
Fractured humeral head or shaft (Figure 4.8)	Immobilization in 'U' slab POP Follow up fracture clinic Pain relief	Application of 'U' slab POP Collar and cuff
Rotator cuff sprain	Referral for physiotherapy Or advice on gradual mobilization Pain relief	Sling/collar and cuff
Adhesive capsulitis 'Frozen shoulder'	A chronic condition that may benefit from physiotherapy once pain is controlled but can continue for 2–3 years with varying symptoms	Collar and cuff only in acute phase of pain

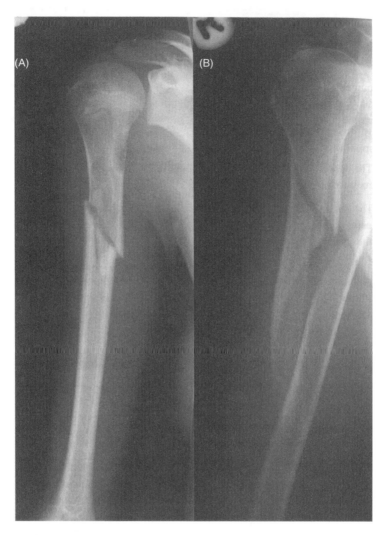

Note: Much more information is provided by lateral view in terms of fragmentation, separation and angulation. Note also that the elbow is not on these films.

Source: Begg (2005)

Figure 4.8 (A) AP (B) lateral views of a spiral fracture of the humerus

Red flags

- Reduced ROM suggesting possible fracture/dislocation
- Altered sensation distally suggesting nerve damage
- Reduced distal pulses

- Fractured scapula can be indicative of more serious chest/abdominal injury.

The foot

History

Injuries to the foot can occur due to inversion or eversion of the ankle, but are more often related to their positional vulnerability by more common mechanisms of injury such as crush, hyper-dorsi/plantar flexion, internal/external rotation or the force of bearing total body weight. The toes are particularly vulnerable and, despite their relative size, the pain produced from fracture can greatly impair mobility.

Delayed presentations, days or week after injury, should be treated with an element of caution as not all fractures prevent weight bearing. Subtle clues such as walking with a slight limp or a point of specific pain in the foot, possibly accompanied by redness or bruising, should be investigated further.

Examination findings/relevant anatomy

Look
Deformity is obviously noticed in the toe areas by comparing the right to the left or in the inward to outward rotation caused by fracture or dislocation.

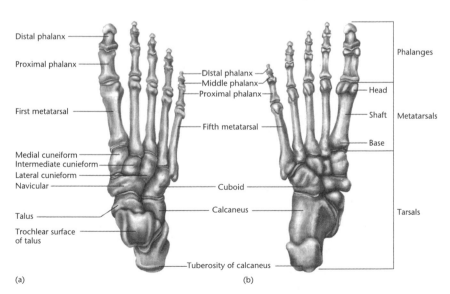

Source: Saladin (2005) (Reproduced with permission)

Figure 4.9 The right foot (a) superior (dorsal) view and (b) inferior (plantar) view

Deformity of the metatarsal may be obvious due to development of tissue swelling that is exacerbated by the effects of gravity in the initial phase after injury.

Bruising around the toes without obvious tenderness can be suggestive of injury in the forefoot and is a common finding in delayed presentations and is often the reason the patient presents.

Bleeding under the toe nails (subungal haematoma) is most common in the great toe and will be caused by some form of crush injury. The condition can produce an immense amount of discomfort for a patient who may present some hours after the injury as the evolving haematoma applies pressure to the nerves of the damaged nail bed. The pain experienced may appear disproportionate to the actual visual appearance of the injury, but a fracture of the underlying bone should be excluded and release of the pressure caused by the haematoma by trephining will provide immediate pain relief.

Areas of erythema (redness) should be noted but can relate to the normal rubbing effect of footwear, a factor that may be mirrored in the other limb. Erythema is a common sign following recent soft tissue injury and relates to the inflammatory process. Erythema around an isolated joint is a significant sign and will be addressed in the next paragraph.

Feel

Adopting the approach of the Ottawa ankle rules (Stiell et al. 1992) (Figure 4.10) is a useful tool in identifying bony injury to the fifth metatarsal base and the navicular. Commence palpation by establishing the focus of the patient's pain; initially avoiding that area will prevent misleading findings as the patient tenses in anticipation. Particular attention should be made to palpating bones of the foot in a linear fashion including the tarsal bones of the midfoot and the lengths of metatarsals and toes.

The assessment of circulation and reduced sensation can be complicated by the recent application of ice packs, soft tissue swelling and pre-existing conditions such as peripheral vascular disease and peripheral neuropathies. Pedal pulses must be noted in the acute phase after trauma with capillary refill assessed in at least the great toe.

Comparing sensation with the right and left sides will establish any deficit, which can be subjective due to the patient's perception when in pain. Often the patient will describe the toes as feeling sleepy or different.

Move

Movements of the foot can be inhibited due to pain. Acutely a minimum level that can be expected includes dorsi and plantar flexion, inversion and eversion, and whether the patient can weight bear.

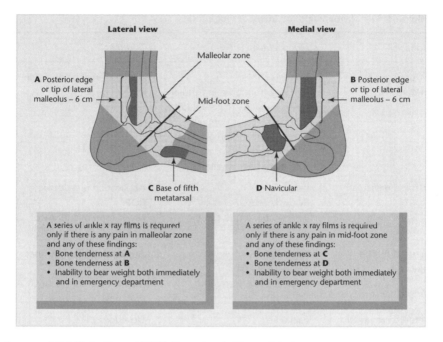

Lateral view

Medial view

Malleolar zone

A Posterior edge
or tip of lateral
malleolus – 6 cm

B Posterior edge
or tip of lateral
malleolus – 6 cm

Mid-foot zone

C Base of fifth
metatarsal

D Navicular

A series of ankle x ray films is required
only if there is any pain in malleolar zone
and any of these findings:
• Bone tenderness at **A**
• Bone tenderness at **B**
• Inability to bear weight both immediately
 and in emergency department

A series of ankle x ray films is required
only if there is any pain in mid-foot zone
and any of these findings:
• Bone tenderness at **C**
• Bone tenderness at **D**
• Inability to bear weight both immediately
 and in emergency department

Source: *British Medical Journal* (2003) (Reproduced with permission)

Figure 4.10 Ottawa ankle rules

Initial intervention

As with the ankle, pain should be addressed, in the acute phase after injury simple methods of elevation of the foot to hip height or higher, cryotherapy and the use of crutches can reduce the level of pain experienced.

Wounds to the foot should be cleaned at the time of initial assessment to minimize the exposure to contaminants potentially containing tetanus spores.

An X-ray can be considered for excluding soft tissue foreign bodies or foot views if bony tenderness is suspected.

Red flags

Cold/mottled appearance of the foot is suggestive of inadequate perfusion. A fall from a significant height, landing on their feet, transferred force injuries to knees, hips, back or neck and calcaneum fractures should be excluded. Pain in the foot without injury, with a loss of sensation can originate from a problem with the back involving the lumber spine region.

Table 4.4 Management and treatment of foot injuries

Diagnosis	Management	Treatment
Fracture base 5th metatarsal	Pain relief Can vary from double tubular elastic bandage to below knee, POP back slab or fibre glass 'bootie', depending on pain and swelling Referral to fracture clinic	Application of below-knee POP Crutches
Fractured navicular	Pain relief Below-knee POP Referral to fracture clinic	Application of below-knee POP Measurement and use of crutches
Fractured shaft of metatarsal	Pain relief Below-knee POP Referral to fracture clinic	Application of below-knee POP Measurement and use of crutches
Fractured calcanuem (Figure 4.11)	Pain relief In the acute phase referred to orthopaedics as often admitted for bed rest to monitor soft tissue swelling and the possible development of compartment syndrome caused by damage to the medial arteries supplying the heel	Elevation Ice packs
Fractured great toe	Pain relief Non-weight bearing on crutches or plaster 'bootie', depending on pain Referral to fracture clinic	Application plaster 'bootie' Measurement and use of crutches
Fractured toes	Diagnosis of fracture made by clinical examination, X-ray only indicated if deformity present Neighbour strapping Advise on analgesia, supportive footwear and walking normally rather than limping	Application neighbour strapping

Diagnosis	Management	Treatment
Stress fracture metatarsals	Diagnosis based on clinical findings rather than on X-ray Referral to fracture clinic Advised to rest Non-weight bearing if pain severe or limping, application below-knee POP	Measurement and use of crutches Possible application below-knee POP
Plantar fasciitis	NSAIDs recommended Advised on initial rest and exercises directed towards strengthening and supporting arch of the foot	Knowledge of physiotherapy exercises recommended
Gout (most common MTPJ great toe)	Diagnosis confirmed with blood test confirming raised uric levels Directed towards adequate pain relief in acute phase Follow up with general practitioner and commenced on xanthine-oxidase inhibitor if condition becomes recurrent	Recognition of condition and severity of pain at initial assessment

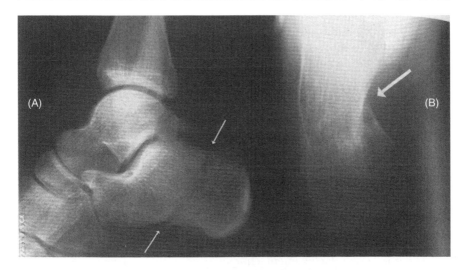

Note: The arrow points to the fracture on the concave or medial side.

Source: Begg (2005)

Figure 4.11 (A) Lateral view showing fracture of calcaneum (arrows) (B) axial view

The ankle

History

Ankle injuries are a common presentation to EDs, with inversion being the most frequent mechanism of injury. Accounts of hearing a clicking or cracking noise coming from the ankle at the time of injury is usually due to tearing of ligaments rather than the snapping of bones. Although rare and often associated with significant lateral or medial force, fracture dislocations of the ankle must be identified promptly to prevent permanent disability for the patient. Immediate recognition and intervention by the practitioner of this condition are vital to ensure that the ankle joint is manipulated back into position, to restore optimum circulation, sensation and function, before an X-ray is taken.

Other common mechanisms of injury to the ankle include:

- Hyperplantar flexion, caused by catching the forefoot when ascending or descending stairs causing excessive stretching of anterior muscles and ligaments leading to sprain or avulsions of the talus.
- Rotation of the ankle in an internal or external movement can cause a spiral fracture to the distal fibula (lateral malleolus), e.g., football studs catching in turf.
- Sudden tightening of the gastrocnemius muscles in the calf when making a move to run forwards can result in an Achilles gastrocnemius rupture. The patient may describe a sensation of being kicked or shot in the back of the ankle or calf.

Examination findings/relevant anatomy

Look

Abnormal appearance (deformity) of the ankle could suggest a serious injury, for example, fracture dislocation (Potts fracture), immense, diffuse or widespread soft tissue swelling around the ankle can be deceptive in masking the definition of normal anatomical landmarks (red flag). Comparing the right ankle with the left assists with assessment of the severity of the presentation and excludes normal variants, e.g., oedematous ankles due to poor venous return.

The most common ankle sprain following inversion injury will affect the anterior talofibular ligament characterized with localized swelling seen over the anterior aspect of the distal fibular.

Localized swelling isolated to the posterior aspect of the ankle can be indicative of Achilles full or partial rupture.

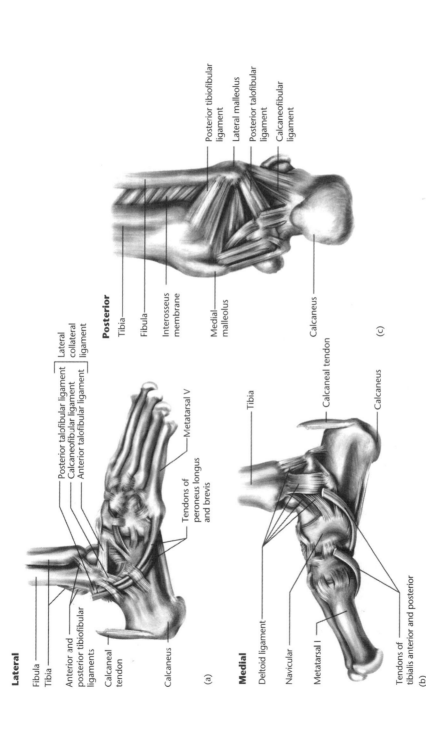

Lateral

Fibula
Tibia
Anterior and posterior tibiofibular ligaments
Calcaneal tendon
Calcaneus

Posterior talofibular ligament
Calcaneofibular ligament — Lateral collateral ligament
Anterior talofibular ligament

Tendons of peroneus longus and brevis
Metatarsal V

(a)

Medial

Deltoid ligament
Navicular
Metatarsal I
Tendons of tibialis anterior and posterior

Tibia
Calcaneal tendon
Calcaneus

(b)

Posterior

Tibia
Fibula
Interosseus membrane
Medial malleolus

Posterior tibiofibular ligament
Lateral malleolus
Posterior talofibular ligament
Calcaneofibular ligament

Calcaneus

(c)

Source: Saladin (2005) (Reproduced with permission)

Figure 4.12 The talocrural (ankle) joint and ligaments of the right foot: (a) lateral view; (b) medial view; (c) posterior view

Immediate bruising can be suggestive of significant joint disruption due to haematoma formation or fracture, late onset bruising is synonymous with ligament sprains.

Feel

Adopting a systematic approach such as the 'Ottawa ankle rules' will enable red flag signs of joint instability or dislocation to be identified. The original concept was formulated to identify bony tenderness indicating fracture in specific sites, and to reduce the volume of unnecessary X-rays or inappropriate views being ordered. It is a method that is internationally recognized and can be modified for the use of practitioner to include palpation of the medial and lateral ligaments of the ankle, to exclude the presence of soft tissue tenderness that could indicate ankle joint dislocation/instability (red flag).

Move

In the acute presentation, assessment of ankle injury movement can be problematic due to pain, so pain scoring with review after the administration of analgesia can enhance secondary examination. The ability to weight bear accompanied by the presence of flexion and extension of the foot is the minimum requirement for the purpose of initial assessment, with weight bearing being a feature of Ottawa rules assessment.

Initial intervention

Pain should be addressed with analgesia and adjuncts such as elevation of the ankle to hip height or higher.

If an unstable ankle is identified, the use of a splint will immobilize the injury, preventing further injury, and reducing pain. The patient should remain non-weight bearing until fully assessed reducing further injury.

Application of an ice pack (cryotherapy) for 15–20 minutes on initial presentation can be of great benefit to minimize swelling, but be aware of the following:

- Prolonged application of an ice pack or direct cold contact with the skin can lead to ice burns, so to aid conduction and protect the skin, cover the pack with a clean, damp disposable cloth and inform the patient of the time limitation.
- Crushed ice or frozen peas mould better to the irregular shape of an ankle.
- Excessive movement of the ice pack can be reduced by the light application of tape or bandage.

Once these issues have been addressed, the ordering of an X-ray can be considered, using the Ottawa rules criteria, always seek a senior opinion if unsure.

Table 4.5 Management and treatment of ankle injuries

Diagnosis	Management	Treatment
Ligament sprains: Grade 1 – Minor tears of the ligaments but no instability or laxity	Pain relief Ice, elevation, early mobilization Referral physiotherapy an option Generally a movement away from use of double layer tubular bandage (Cooper et al. 1997)	Advice on care of ankle sprain Refer to local policy Strapping Application of double layer tubular bandage
Grade 2 – Ankle joint stable but tears to ligament sufficient to cause laxity	Pain relief Ice, elevation, Follow up either to physiotherapy or fracture clinic Non-weight bearing crutches Below-knee POP back slab for pain relief if in obvious discomfort, with its use kept to a minimum time possible	Advice on care of ankle sprain Application below-knee POP back slab Measurement and use of crutches
Grade 3 – Tears to ligament fibres so severe that the laxity means the joint is totally unstable	Pain relief Ice, elevation, Below-knee POP back slab Referral to on-call orthopaedic team	Application below-knee POP back slab Elevation greater that hip level
Rupture of Achilles tendon (total or partial)	Pain relief Ice, elevation Referral to on-call orthopaedic +/– diagnostic ultra sound Treatment options vary from surgical repair to conservative management Below-knee POP back slab Non-weight bearing crutches Managed in equinous POP	Advanced skill of application of equinous POP Measurement and use of crutches if discharged to home
Fractured lateral malleolus Weber A fracture below the ankle joint	Pain relief Ice, elevation, Below-knee POP back slab Non-weight bearing crutches Pain relief	Application below-knee POP back slab Measurement and use of crutches

Diagnosis	Management	Treatment
Weber B fracture at the level of the joint, with the tibiofibular ligaments usually intact	If fracture is displaced referral to on-call orthopaedic team for opinion Otherwise application of below-knee POP back slab Non-weight bearing crutches Follow up in fracture clinic Pain relief Referral to on-call orthopaedic team for possible internal fixation as unstable	Application below-knee POP back slab Measurement and use of crutches
Weber C fracture above the joint level which tears the syndesmotic ligaments	Application of below-knee POP back slab for comfort prior to surgery High elevation to minimize swelling	Application of below-knee POP back slab for comfort prior to surgery High elevation to minimize swelling
Fractured medial and lateral malleolus (Bi-malleolar fracture) +/– Talar shift	Pain relief Referral to on-call orthopaedic team for possible internal fixation as unstable Application of below-knee POP back slab for comfort prior to surgery High elevation to minimize swelling	Application of below knee POP back slab for comfort prior to surgery High elevation to minimize swelling
Dislocation +/– fracture medial and lateral malleolus (Bi-malleolar fracture) also known as Potts fracture	Alert senior colleague This requires urgent manipulation under sedation/pain relief before even considering X-ray Referral to on-call orthopaedic team for internal fixation as grossly unstable Application of below-knee POP back slab for comfort prior to surgery High elevation to minimize swelling	Initially direct to resuscitation area mainly for space and observation during manipulation Assist with manipulation Application of below-knee POP back slab for comfort prior to surgery High elevation to minimize swelling
Septic arthritis	Pain relief Referral to orthopaedic team	

Red flags

Absence of pedal pulses or a delayed capillary refill are significant signs that should be reported to senior colleagues. Cold/mottled appearance of the foot is suggestive of inadequate perfusion. Deformity suggesting dislocation, medial malleolus tenderness and lateral tenderness following injury are suggestive of fracture dislocation requiring urgent manipulation. A hot, swollen ankle joint with severe pain and reduced range of movement should be treated as a possible septic arthritis.

Patients presenting with continued pain, despite a previously normal X-ray, require closer examination and repeat X-rays may reveal a fracture.

The knee

History

Minor knee injuries are a common presentation as a result of a fall. The mechanism of injury will vary from landing directly on the patella with a flexed knee or a force causing a medial or lateral movement resulting in a valgus or varus strain due to the high velocity impact, such as blunt trauma caused by the impact of a car bumper, seen in road traffic accidents.

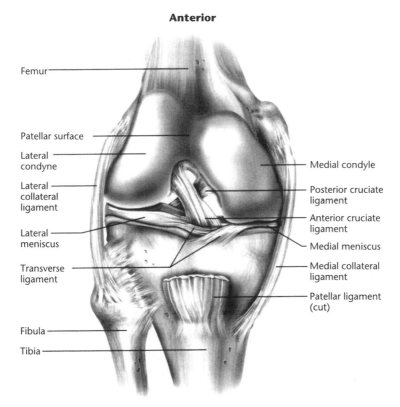

Anterior

Femur

Patellar surface

Lateral condyne

Medial condyle

Lateral collateral ligament

Posterior cruciate ligament

Anterior cruciate ligament

Lateral meniscus

Medial meniscus

Transverse ligament

Medial collateral ligament

Patellar ligament (cut)

Fibula

Tibia

Note: Anterior view of structures in the joint cavity of the right knee

Source: Saladin (2005) (Reproduced with permission)

Figure 4.13 The knee joint

Features include:

- Sudden onset of swelling (effusion) = anterior cruciate ligament (ACL) or posterior cruciate ligament (PCL) injury causing bleeding into joint
- Popping sounds at the time of injury = ACL/PCL rupture
- Painless giving way leading to falling = ACL/PCL rupture, collateral ligament rupture
- Locking = tear meniscus (shock absorber)
- Hot, inflamed tender joint = septic arthritis.

Examination findings/relevant anatomy

Look
Abnormal appearance or deformity to the knee should raise suspicion of serious injury, but is unlikely to appear without more significant signs such as pain, e.g., dislocated patella (common), dislocated knee joint (rare).

Generalized swelling over the anterior aspect of the knee can lead to a lack of contour of the patella and is indicative of a significant build-up of synovial fluid or blood suggesting effusion or haemoarthrosis.

Localized swelling relates to direct blunt force to the area and is commonly seen over the distal end of the patella. Localized bruising in the initial period is not unusual, If seen over the posterior aspect of the knee without direct trauma is highly suggestive of a ruptured baker's cyst.

Feel
Examination of a patient's knee can be difficult, often due to the pain, resulting in the patient tensing their quadriceps muscles thus restricting flexion or extension movements. For initial assessment purposes it is pertinent to exclude pain above and below the knee joint, e.g., hip and ankle. Tenderness over the following sites would be suggestive of either soft tissue or bony injury:

- Patella
- Proximal tibia (tibial plateau fracture)
- Proximal fibula (fractured proximal fibula, need to exclude rotating force causing fracture distal fibula and nerve damage)
- Lateral/medial joint line tenderness (suggestive of menicial tear)
- Crepitus over patella (degenerative changes, e.g., osteoarthritis)
- Widespread heat and tenderness (consider septic arthritis) producing pain on palpation.

As with the ankle, the Ottawa knee rules are a useful tool in establishing whether an X-ray is indicated.

Move

The ability to weight bear, flex, extend or straight leg raise is the minimum requirement for any initial assessment of a knee. Early recognition of the following findings will highlight most of the major red flag conditions:

1 Non-weight bearing:

- Dislocation
- Fractured tibial plateau
- Fractured femur
- ACL/PCL instability/rupture
- MCL/LCL instability/rupture
- Pain

2 Reduced flexion:

- Could be due to pain

3 Reduced extension:

- Tear to meniscus
- Effusion

4 Unable to straight leg raise:

- Ruptured patella tendon.

Initial intervention

Pain assessment and relief should be a priority in order to enhance the patient's comfort and improve the examination experience.

Immobilizing the knee in a splint to aid pain relief is often impractical; the use of non-weight bearing on crutches or a wheelchair can be useful.

Elevation of the injury in the initial stages should be encouraged, with the support of a pillow or blanket to relieve muscle tension/spasm that occurs when a patient is in pain.

Table 4.6 Management and treatment of knee injuries

Diagnosis	Management	Treatment
Fractured patella	Pain relief Discuss management with on-call orthopaedic team Application of POP cylinder cast Non-weight bearing crutches Elevation	Application of POP cylinder cast Measurement and use of crutches

Diagnosis	Management	Treatment
Rupture of patella tendon	Pain relief Discuss management with on-call orthopaedic team Application of POP cylinder cast Non-weight-bearing crutches Elevation	Application of POP cylinder cast Measurement and use of crutches
Medial or lateral collateral ligament sprain	Providing no laxity, refer for physiotherapy If limping, partial weight bearing on crutches Rest, ice, elevation Referral to physiotherapy an option Generally a movement away from use of double layer tubular bandage (Cooper et al. 1997) but from experience the author has noticed patients comment on the support they feel with one on	Advise on care of soft tissue injury Measurement and use of crutches
Medial or lateral meniscus tear	Pain relief Rest, ice, elevation Partial weight-bearing in crutches if limping Refer to physiotherapy, if not improving may require orthopaedic referral	Advise on care of soft tissue injury Measurement and use of crutches
Locked knee	Pain relief Urgent referral to on-call orthopaedic team	
Anterior or posterior cruciate ligament rupture	Pain relief Discuss with orthopaedic on call Admission for repair under general anaesthetic POP full leg back slab for pain relief prior to surgery High elevation	Application of POP full leg back slab High elevation
Fractured tibial plateau (Figure 4.14)	Pain relief Refer to on-call orthopaedic team Admission for internal fixation under general anaesthetic POP full leg back slab for pain relief prior to surgery High elevation	Application of POP full leg back slab High elevation
Tense effusion Possible haemoarthrosis	Pain relief Discuss with on-call orthopaedic team which may lead to aspiration under strict aseptic technique Application of POP, cricket pad splint or Robert Jones bandage depending on cause of effusion	Assist with knee aspiration

Diagnosis	Management	Treatment
Fractured fibula	Pain relief Will depend on type of fracture but may include application of full leg POP back slab and non-weight-bearing crutches	Application of POP full leg back slab Measurement and use of crutches
Pre-patella bursitis	Pain relief Exclude infection Refrain from activity triggering inflammation NSAIDS	

Red flags

Deformed patella indicates dislocation, requiring manipulation under sedation. Tenderness over proximal tibia indicates tibial plateau fracture requiring internal fixation. Inability to straight leg raise, possible ruptured patella tendon.

Septic arthritis is a rare condition characterized by severe pain, heat and swelling in a joint with loss of function, caused by infection. This is a medical emergency as sepsis is possible. A true locked knee requires urgent referral to the orthopaedic team.

Wound assessment

History

Emergency practitioners encounter wounds on a daily basis; it is an area that many junior practitioners identify as an area of weakness when applying theory to practice. Building expertise in this area should start with information gathering at initial assessment in order to establish priorities of care by using the questioning framework of, Who? What? When? How? Where?

How
Establishing the mechanism of injury is vital:

- Cut – from a medico-legal stance this implies a straight-edged incised wound often caused by a sharp edge such as broken glass or the blade of a knife.
- Laceration – from a medico-legal stance suggests a jagged-edged wound caused by blunt trauma. Generally laceration is used to refer to deep or partial thickness separation of skin layers.
- Abrasion – skin loss caused by friction, can be superficial, partial or full thickness

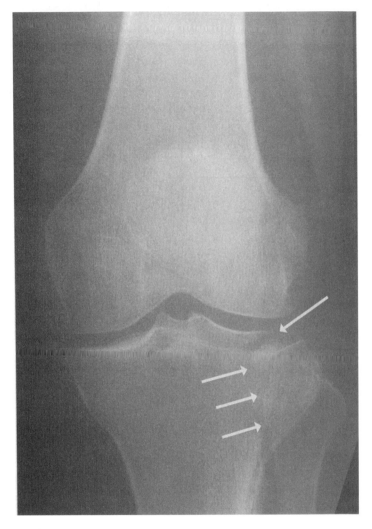

Source: Begg (2005)

Figure 4.14 A depressed fracture of the lateral tibial plateau (arrows)

- Flap – implies oblique entry to the skin creating the wound, which can be deep or superficial, causing damage to the tissues.
- Puncture – referring to a penetrating injury at a concentrated point in the skin. The significance is that it may appear innocent to the naked eye, the potential risk for infection is high, as the object may have driven bacteria deep within the tissues providing the perfect warm, moist environment for bacterial proliferation.

- Bites – whether human or animal in origin, infection is a common complication and negates the initial closure of the wound.
- Crush – the skin can split, can cause a laceration to the underlying nail bed.
- Burn (or thermal injury) – direct contact with flame, hot water, steam, sunlight, chemicals, radiation, extreme cold or friction. The duration and nature of the exposure will dictate the depth of damage to the dermis and epidermis and is classified as being either superficial, partial thickness or full thickness.
- Abscess – a localized collection of tissue debris and lymphocytes as a direct result of widespread tissue death due to infection, often related to sebaceous cysts, commonly known as pus. While the abscess develops, it produces increasing pain, due to the accompanying soft tissue inflammation and swelling. As the pressure builds, the enclosed collection can break through the skin surface allowing the cystic and pus contents to discharge, leaving a cavity that will eventually heal from the base of the wound to the surface of the skin through granulation.

Who

- Occupation – whether a concert pianist, chef, labourer or in retirement can influence the significance of the wound on daily activities and modifications that can be made to treatment to accommodate that, e.g., labourers are often self-employed, so do not receive sick pay and hence return to work immediately following injury despite medical warnings to the contrary. In this situation it would be pertinent to secure dressings more robustly and provide the patient with additional dressings to allow more frequent changes of dirty ones.
- Age – healing can be impaired in the elderly due to poor circulation.
- Medical conditions – diabetic patients are more at risk from developing infections due to the increased sugar content in their blood, poor distal blood supply and diabetic neuropathy.
- Ethnicity – keloid scarring can be a complication to wound healing in patients with black skin. Following burn injuries Caucasian skins become more sensitive to sunlight requiring a higher sun cream protection factor.
- Despite most Western countries having health policies requiring children to be vaccinated against tetanus, tetanus vaccination status should always be established.

What

What part of the body was affected can influence ongoing treatment priorities:

- Blunt trauma to the head resulting in a wound and formation of a haematoma could require initial cleansing and application of pressure, followed by neurological observations.

- Wounds to the pre-tibial area occur frequently in the elderly, commonly sustained on the edge of steps when climbing on a bus, taxi or escalator. Due to reduced circulation, infection and delayed healing are common.

When

Bruising and swelling can initially complicate the assessment process. Blood loss at the time of injury should be estimated and first aid measures identified.

Delayed presentation of wounds can inhibit positive outcomes of treatment when lack of cleansing increases the risk of infection. Wound edges can swell during the inflammatory process and scarring can occur. Local infection policies may specify that after a certain time period wounds should not be sutured, e.g., 12 hrs. In practice the clinician can evaluate on an individual basis as scarring can be greatly reduced by drawing wound edges closer. The wound edges may not totally unite, allowing any excessive serous or bloody exudate to drain and reduce the production of collagen fibres that cause scarring (improving the cosmetic result). In this situation treatment options would be discussed with the patient, prophylactic antibiotics considered and the patient warned of the risks and implications of scarring or infection.

Where

Understanding the environment where the injury took place is vital in assessing the current risks for effective patient outcomes. A wound sustained on a farm contaminated with soil or manure would be a high risk for tetanus as well as infection compared to the low risk of a cut sustained with a clean kitchen knife.

Location can be significant if the injury was sustained in a country where indigenous hazards to that local area may be unfamiliar to the assessor, i.e., burrowing skin worms found in Africa, or embedded coral spines in tropical seas.

Examination findings/relevant anatomy

When examining a wound, documenting the following significant findings immediately identifies the priorities for ongoing care management.

Look

- What type of wound is this? E.g., cut, abrasion, puncture, crush.
- How long is the wound and what shape is it? Measuring the wound is helpful in expressing the severity of the injury.
- Is the wound clean? The wound may be contaminated with dirt, soil or foreign bodies such as wood or fibres of clothing.

- How deep is the wound? Defined as: deep, partial thickness, superficial.
- Is there any evidence of active bleeding? Suggesting volume, severity of blood loss and whether there is arterial or venous vessel damage.
- Are the wound edges opposed or gaping? Are other structures visible? E.g., fat layer, tendons, bone, muscles.
- Are those structures damaged? A full or partial cut to the tendon sheath, or fascia of a muscle.
- Is there swelling, redness or discharge? Suggesting infection or soft tissue trauma.
- Does the appearance of the wound fit with the mechanism of injury? Occasionally a patient may withhold facts about their injury, because of embarrassment or illegal activity. Confidentiality must be respected and expressed to the patient, so that their care is not compromised, even if the true cause of the injury is not disclosed.

Feel

Sensation should always be considered when assessing any patient with a minor injury, taking particular significance in an incised wound, where nerves may be cut. It is not unusual for patients to experience a loss of sensation in the immediate skin area approximately 5mm from the wound edge, when nerve endings providing local sensation, are damaged. A loss of sensation distal to the cut, e.g., a cut to the proximal end of a finger may cause the patient to totally or partially lose sensation to the whole skin area distal to the cut, suggesting a severing of the digital nerve, which can be repaired by plastic surgeons if treated within the first 2–3 days after injury. The minimum standard for initially assessing sensation to the fingers should involve touching each finger in turn, with comparison with the finger on the other, unaffected, hand. In other parts of the body it can be achieved by touching the skin of the patient in the distal part of the affected limb. The patient may have total numbness, more often they will describe a sensation of the digit feeling different or sleepy, which may be indicative of a severed nerve injury or may be neuropraxia.

Move

Generally an isolated wound would not be the direct mechanical cause for preventing movement of a limb. An example of a direct cause would be a cut to an underlying structure, such as tendons, which would reduce movements such as flexion or extension in a finger, depending on the location. Pain commonly causes restriction to movement, in particular for wounds over joints like the knee and elbow, which during flexion will pull on wound edges and stimulate exposed sensory nerve endings. Abrasions in the same areas can produce the same effect, especially if a wide area is affected where the scab formation has become dried and cracked. Soft tissue swelling and inflammation from an abscess such as a peri-anal abscess can restrict walking or sitting.

Initial intervention

Cleaning wounds during initial assessment is one of the most undervalued and underutilized interventions in emergency wound care management. Time pressures can contribute to this, although cleaning the wound is paramount to efficient wound examination, place the wound under running tapwater to remove skin contaminants.

With burns the priority is to remove excessive heat from the damaged tissues: the most effective method is to expose the affected area to running, cold tapwater.

Diagnosis

Care diagnosis and initial assessment are very closely interlinked, the practitioner making the initial assessment could treat the patient and discharge them from triage.

Wound care management should be guided by the following practice guidelines for wound closure:

- All wounds should be thoroughly cleansed by irrigation.
- Wound closure decisions should be made on the most effective method for opposing wound edges, minimizing additional trauma to the skin.
- Steri-strips can only be effectively used on non-actively bleeding wounds where very little tension is needed to unite wound edges.
- Tissue adhesives should be used with caution. Protect the eyes with saline soaks if applying in the eyebrow region and lay the patient supine. The wound edges should unite without tension and there should be no gaps that allow glue to seep to the wound base, as ulcer formation is possible, so remove the plug of glue.
- If you are unable to clearly view the base of the wound, then before closure the wound must be fully explored possibly under local anaesthetic to ensure all underlying structures are intact.
- Pre-tibial lacerations should never be sutured. Occasionally a few anchoring sutures may be used; steri-strips are preferred to minimize damage to delicate tissues.
- Human or animal bite wounds should not be closed at the time of injury.
- Following incision and drainage of an abscess, wound edges should be kept apart to allow for further drainage of exudates. Dressing choices

such as some alginates appear to reduce pain experienced by the patient during removal.

Red flags

- Loss of sensation
- Active bleeding
- Retained FB
- Infection
- Diabetics
- Elderly steroid therapy
- MRSA
- Wounds sustained in environments that the practitioner is unfamiliar with e.g. spider bites, coral foreign bodies, burrowing worms, frost bite.

Minor illness

Minor illness is a vast subject, often affecting many physiological processes that culminate in a collection of varying signs and symptoms. For the purpose of this section the most frequently occurring conditions will be discussed, including the more serious differential diagnosis that the practitioner should exclude before deciding on a treatment priority. This will be presented in a grid format (Table 4.7). It is important to recognize that signs and symptoms may present in isolation, affecting one structure, e.g., deafness due to wax build-up, or in a myriad collection as in cold or flu. The health professional must sort through and critically analyse all data in order to discover the cause, as well as the patient's agenda and medical priority.

The inexperienced practitioner will develop their own routine in arriving at the decision-making stage, and initially this can be achieved by following the logical process outlined in the grid.

Questions to assist with history taking

- Duration of symptoms?
- Chronological order how symptoms developed?
- Reason for presentation?
- Remedies already tried?
- Have they had this problem before and how frequently does it occur?
- Has anyone else you know been ill with the same complaint?
- Any recent overseas travel?

Table 4.7 Minor illness reference chart

Symptom	History	Examination findings of relevant anatomy	Initial intervention	Diagnosis	Treatment	Skill	Red flags
Sore throat	Pain in throat made worse by swallowing Usually presents after 3–4 days Related to cold symptoms	Swollen tonsils bilaterally Pus in crypts Inflammation pharynx Pyrexia (Figure 4.15)	Pain relief	Bacterial tonsillitis Viral tonsillitis Peritonsillar abscess (quinsy) (Figure 4.15) Pharyngitis Mononucleosis FB	Oral antibiotics such as penicillin/ erythromycin	Examination of throat using auroscope and tongue depressor	Peritonsillar abscess (quinsy) Obstruction Possibly cancer in elderly Gonococcal pharyngitis
Unable to swallow saliva (adult)	Worsening sore throat Pooling of saliva in mouth	Sore throat Unilateral swelling pharynx Pyrexia	Nil by mouth Urgent priority due to possible compromised airway	Peritonsillar abscess (quinsy) Obstruction	Referral to ENT specialist for I+D of abscess/IV antibiotics	Monitor airway O2 sat Respiratory rate O2 therapy	Foreign body Severe allergic reaction
Unable to swallow saliva (child)	Sore throat in child leading to drooling	Do not look into airway Drooling, sit leaning forward, preferring to spit out saliva rather than swallow Stridor	Urgent priority due to possible compromised airway	Epiglottitis	IV antibiotics administration	Reassurance Monitor airway O2 sat Respiratory rate O2 therapy	Foreign body Severe allergic reaction

Symptom	Presentation	Examination findings		Diagnosis	Management	Test quality of hearing	Complications
Deafness	Gradual/sudden Onset of reduced or loss hearing in one ear Painful or painless	External auditory canal blocked with wax deposits often obscuring vision of tympanic membrane (ear drum)	Pain relief to facilitate ear examination	Wax build-up Otitis media	Application of wax softener to affected ear for 5 days, then ear syringing by practice nurse	Test quality of hearing by seeing if patient can hear you rubbing your fingers together by the affected ear Examination of ears using auroscope, viewing unaffected ear first	Perforated ear drum from using cotton buds to dislodge wax Foreign body Middle ear effusion
Painful ear	Complication of sore throat when infection ascends Eustachian tube	Painful ear lobe on palpation Ear drum inflamed, Opaque, bulging	Pain relief	Otitis media	Pain relief oral antibiotics	Examination of ears using auroscope viewing unaffected ear first	Perforation Pharyngitis
	Increasing itching or soreness in ear canal prior to developing pain. Can be related to wax build-up or trauma such as use of cotton bud causing abrasion to surface ear canal	Ear canal moist with wax, serous and tissue debris. In severe cases ear canal narrowed due to infection restricting view of ear drum	Pain relief	Otitis externa	Pain relief Antibiotic drops Severe cases referred to ENT for ear toilet and/insertion antibiotic wick		Recurrence mastoiditis

Table 4.7—continued

Symptom	History	Examination findings of relevant anatomy	Initial intervention	Diagnosis	Treatment	Skill	Red flags
Discharging ear	Complication of Otitis media infection leading to sudden severe sharp pain in one ear. Can be made worse by air travel	Pus discharge visible in ear canal and perforation of ear drum	Analgesia	Otitis media Perforated ear drum	Antibiotics Analgesia Review GP to ensure perforation healing	Examination of ears using auroscope, viewing unaffected ear first	Otitis media cellulitis
	Itching ears that have become increasingly sore and now experiencing clear serous discharge			Otitis externa	Pain relief Antibiotic drops Severe cases referred to ENT for ear toilet and/insertion antibiotic wick	Examination of ears using auroscope, viewing unaffected ear first	Otitis media Mastoiditis Cholesteatoma Eczema Psoriasis
Itchy ears	Increasing itching or soreness in ear canal prior to development pain. Can be related to wax build-up or trauma such as use of cotton bud causing abrasion to surface ear canal	Ear canal moist with wax, serous and tissue debris In severe cases ear canal narrowed due to infection restricting view of ear drum	Pain Relief	Otitis externa Wax build-up Eczema	Pain relief Antibiotic drops Severe cases referred to ENT for ear toilet and/insertion antibiotic wick	Examination of ears using auroscope	Exclude foreign body Otitis media Mastoiditis Cholesteatoma Eczema Psoriasis
	Gradual onset of dry, itchy, flaking skin in ear canal extending over ear lobe	Erythematous dry flaking/serous seeping skin in ear canal possibly affecting ear lobe	Nil indicated but pain relief or anti-histamine if patient distressed		Use wax softeners once infection subsides with education over ear care Topical steroid antibiotics if infected		Cellulitis Otitis externa

Itchy eyes	Increasing irritation and watering of both eyes following exposure to an irritant such as pollen or make-up	Eyelids may be red, swollen Excessive watering Conjunctiva will appear swollen	Check visual acuity Application of cool compress	Allergic Conjunctivitis	Oral antihistamine Avoid suspected irritant. Return should condition worsen	Visual acuity Preliminary eye examination	Orbital cellulitis Reduced visual acuity
	Increasing irritation in one or both eyes with soreness and rough sensation when blinking Often waking from sleep with crusty discharge May find bright lights worsen their discomfort Recent contact with a person with conjunctivitis	Lids may be swollen with crusty or mucus-like discharge Conjunctiva appears inflamed	Check visual acuity	Bacterial Conjunctivitis	Antibiotics drops Advise on avoiding hand hygiene and preventing cross-infection	Application of eye drops	Chlamydia Immuno-suppression
	Long-standing sore itchy eyes	Eyelids appear inflamed along line of eyelashes with minute specs dry skin or ulceration around the hair follicle	History taking should exclude any recent eye trauma	Blepharitis	Antibiotics if infected Advise lid hygiene Treatment options directed towards lid cleaning and lubrication	Application of drops and eye lid hygiene	Rosacea
Discharging eyes	Increasing irritation in one or both eyes with soreness and rough sensation when blinking Often waking from sleep with crusty discharge	Lids may be swollen with crusty or mucus-like discharge Conjunctiva appears inflamed	Check visual acuity	Bacterial Conjunctivitis	Antibiotic drops – advice on hand hygiene and preventing cross-infection	Application of eye drops	Chlamydia Immuno-suppression

Table 4.7—continued

Symptom	History	Examination findings of relevant anatomy	Initial intervention	Diagnosis	Treatment	Skill	Red flags
Rhinitis	A combination of sneezing, nasal blockage/irritation	Increased nasal secretions Nasal mucosa swollen and inflamed Patient may appear tired with watering eyes	Reduce exposure to other patients and staff until diagnosis confirmed	Viral illness (common cold) Bacterial Allergy	Patient advised on rest, fluids, regular Paracetamol to relieve pain and fever Directed towards treating source of infection – tonsillitis, sinusitis or chest Antihistamine oral or nasal spray Avoid irritant	Advice directed towards temporarily adapting lifestyle	Exclude history foreign body or recent facial/head trauma Avian flu Meningitis

Symptom	Clinical features		Diagnosis/Notes	Treatment	Advanced skills	Differential diagnoses
Facial pain	Recent URTI Purulent mucus on blowing nose Frontal headache with pain around forehead and nose that worsens on leaning forward Sense of smell reduced Sinus area tender on palpation Nasal passages congested with purulent mucus Patient appears in discomfort	Offer analgesia and antipyretic	Sinusitis	Possibly antibiotics Analgesia Topical decongestants	Advice on steam inhalations	Orbital abscess Meningitis
Facial swelling/ tenderness	Pyrexia Usually develops over 2 days with pyrexia leading to painful/sore swelling around the jaw and parotid glands Extreme pyrexia Marked facial swelling around the jaw line extending to the ears		Mumps is classified as a Health Department notifiable disease	Advice on rest, regular antipyretic and risk of spread through droplet infection	Examination skills to identify specific facial swelling	Orchitis Blocked parotid gland Cellulitis
Cough	Can range from a persistent tickling cough following a cold through to the extremes of productive purulent sputum, pyrexia, night sweats, shortness of breath, haemoptysis, chest pain and weight loss. Differentiation of the significance of those symptoms comes with experience Temperature, pulse, respiration, blood pressure, peak flow, O2 saturation.	Offer analgesia and antipyretic	URTI LRTI	Possible chest X-ray Antibiotics Patient advised on rest, fluids Paracetamol to relieve pain and pyrexia	Advanced history taking skills to exclude red flag conditions	Bronchitis Croup Influenza Pneumonia Pneumothorax Pulmonary embolus TB, Avian flu Carcinoma Asthma Inhaled FB Smoking

- Have they sought the advice of any other health professionals for this problem?
- Have they noticed any rash, stiff neck or raised fever?
- Fever for longer than 1/52?
- Are they experiencing night sweats or weight loss?

 Scenario 4.2 Minor illness assessment

A 19-year-old student presents to the ED with a three-day history of increasing sore throat, fever and runny nose. He presents due to pain on swallowing. On examination he appears flushed, hot to touch with halitosis and is experiencing discomfort when talking.

Vital signs: respiratory rate 16 Pulse 90 BP 110/70 Temperature 38.1

D *Data* (scientific facts): from the initial data collection we can deduce that the patient's airway at present is not compromised, because his respiratory rate is 16 and he is able to speak. The assessor must examine the throat by looking at the tonsils to ensure that a peritonsillar abscess (quinsy) (Figure 4.15) has been excluded; this is a complication of tonsillitis that can potentially lead to an obstructed compromised airway.

A raised temperature of 38 degrees contigrade suggests infection, which may be bacterial or viral in origin, and swelling/tenderness of the cervical and tonsillar lymph glands would support this theory suggesting that there is an increased activity of the patient's immune system through this inflammatory process.

E *Emotions* (intuition): when a patient presents demonstrating obvious discomfort with a severe case of tonsillitis, it is vital that the assessment puts the patient at ease. This can be achieved by demonstrating competence in evaluating their condition and feeding back examination findings with an explanation of their significance to the patient. Anxiety due to pain often exacerbates this condition, so once airway obstruction has been excluded and tonsillitis identified, pain assessment and the administration of analgesia and an antipyretic should be a priority.

A *Advantages*: early identification of quinsy should be followed up by prompt referral and, therefore, intervention by the ear, nose and throat (ENT) specialists to drain the abscess, reducing the risk of obstruction and sepsis.

D *Disadvantages* (differential diagnoses): the assessor should continue to monitor the patient in order to identify any early signs of airway obstruction. In extreme cases the patient may be drooling or pooling their saliva because they are unable to swallow. In this situation the patient prefers to sit leaning forward in order to spit out the excessive saliva.

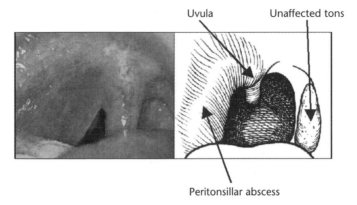

Uvula   Unaffected tons

Peritonsillar abscess

Source: Emedicine at www.emedicinehealth.com/script/main/art.asp?articlekey=58852&pf=3&page=1 (accessed 24 June 2006) Media File 1

Figure 4.15   Peritonsillar abscess (quinsy)

If drooling is seen in young children, never attempt to examine the airway as they may have epiglottis and this could precipitate occlusion of the airway.

Other complications such as meningitis should be considered as a sore throat can be part of a much more serious presentation, with fever, neck rigidity, headache and photophobia forming the greater picture with the classic non-blanching rash.

Glandular fever (mononucleosis) should be considered when the sore throat is prolonged and is especially common in teenagers, confirmed by a blood test.

Conclusion

A solid understanding of both the assessment and treatment of minor injury, and illness, develops a foundation of theoretical knowledge and practical skills that practitioners can build on. These skills are essential to modern practitioners, as the skills of history-taking and physical assessment can be applied to all areas of emergency care. The ability to directly improve the patient experience by delivering care at an expert level is far from an overnight achievement; experiential learning contributes greatly to the individual's professional development and clinical performance. By following, and referring to the information within this chapter, the novice practitioner can begin to develop an array of skills that are both professionally empowering and clearly beneficial to the patient experience.

5 Major trauma: assessment prioritization and initial treatment

Andrew Frazer

Introduction

Major trauma is one of the most exciting and rewarding aspects of emergency care, providing the opportunity to nurse patients with complex acute injuries. It is also an area where errors and omissions may cause significant morbidity and mortality. For this reason a systematic approach to trauma care is necessary, coupled with an understanding of the underlying physiology of acute injuries, in order to recognize and manage potentially life-threatening conditions.

In 1988, the Royal College of Surgeons found deficiencies in trauma care resulting in the avoidable deaths of 33 per cent of a sample of trauma patients admitted to EDs in the UK (Royal College of Surgeons 1988). The organization of trauma education, training and practice in the UK has subsequently developed closely along the lines established by the American College of Surgeons and the Advance Trauma Life Support (ATLS) course. This has undoubtedly improved the ability of doctors to treat acute injury, although there are still significant variations in outcomes for trauma victims across different hospitals. While there are arguments for establishing a UK course, which would be more locally responsive, the established ATLS course provides an international language of trauma care, and it is unlikely that the simple ABCDE approach of the ATLS model could be easily improved. Attendance as an observer on an ATLS course, or better still, as a candidate on an ATNC (Advanced Trauma Nursing Care Course – a five-day course which encompasses the ATLS course with an additional specific nursing focus on trauma) is recommended to embed the knowledge and skills necessary to care for seriously injured patients.

Definition

It is possible to define trauma as any insult to the human body, potentially including isolated psychological trauma. This does not help to differentiate minor and major injuries, however. Technical definitions of 'major' trauma involve complicated scoring mechanisms relating to the severity of anatomical injury, for example, an injury severity score > 15 is defined as 'major trauma' (WHO 2004). While such scoring systems may assist in trauma audit and research, a simpler and more instructive definition for practice describes major trauma as 'life- or limb-threatening injury'.

Prevalence

Trauma is the leading cause of death in the UK in the first four decades of life. There are, therefore, a disproportionate number of younger trauma victims, entailing the enormous socio-economic costs of the loss of many years of productive life and prolonged disability. In the UK blunt trauma is by far the most prevalent mechanism of injury, with road traffic accidents and falls accounting for the majority of injuries. The UK has yet to mirror the unenviable statistics on penetrating trauma from the USA, where gunshot wounds account for around 29,000 deaths per annum.

Organization of trauma care

Most hospitals now manage the seriously injured patient with a 'trauma team' approach. This enables different members of the team to be allocated to specific tasks, which means trauma resuscitation can be undertaken in a concurrent, rather than sequential, manner. Membership of the trauma team varies widely from hospital to hospital, but should include at least those listed in Box 5.1.

In addition to this minimal team, there would ideally be another nurse to care for any relatives who might be present. An additional nurse may prepare equipment for chest drains, obtain analgesia and, as is often forgotten in the bustle of trauma resuscitation, give explanation and comfort to the patient.

There are pre-defined criteria for alerting trauma teams to the imminent arrival of a seriously injured patient. Ideally the team should be activated in advance of the patient's arrival so that assessment and treatment are not delayed – normally a message is relayed to the hospital from the ambulance staff, via the ambulance control centre. Separate criteria for alerting the team pre-hospital and in hospital may apply, but should include the conditions/ mechanisms of injury listed in Box 5.2.

Box 5.1   Trauma team members

Team leader: coordinates team to perform the initial assessment; decides on diagnostic interventions; and formulates definitive plans.

Airway controller (ideally an anaesthetist): establishes clear airway; intubates as required; and ensures the maintenance of spinal immobilization.

General and orthopaedic surgeons: assess and manage specific injuries under the direction of the team leader.

Primary nurse: records information; monitors vital signs; and may undertake cannulation and administer IV fluids.

Secondary nurse: removes patient's clothing; assists primary nurse; may assist anaesthetist in airway control and c-spine immobilization.

A radiographer: to perform X-rays/imaging.

(Adapted from the 'Composition of a typical trauma team', WHO 2004)

Box 5.2   Criteria for trauma team activation

Patients with any of the following:

- Airway compromise: actual or potential
- Signs of pneumothorax
- SpO2 < 90%
- Pulse > 100/minute or systolic blood pressure < 90mmHg (in adults)
- A history of unconsciousness following head injury or GCS < 15
- An incident with 5 or more casualties or involving a fatality
- A high-speed motor vehicle crash, especially where the patient has been ejected from the vehicle
- A penetrating wound other than to the limbs
- Any gunshot wound
- A fall from greater than 8 metres (25 feet)
- A pedestrian or cyclist struck by a vehicle.

(Adapted from the American College of Surgeons 2004)

The trauma team leader should ensure the team is adequately protected from potential pathogens before the patient's arrival. Gloves, plastic aprons and goggles or protective visors are the minimum measures required to adequately reduce the risk of exposure to HIV or hepatitis. Members of the trauma team without these precautions should not approach the patient. Members of the team who are performing the primary survey should also be provided with lead aprons, so that essential X-rays may be obtained without interrupting the patient's management.

The ABCDE approach to initial assessment

The ABCDE approach to trauma care involves recognizing and treating the greatest threat to life first. It would be futile dealing effectively with a patient's significant haemorrhage, for example, if he were unable to breathe because of an unrecognized obstructed airway. The ATLS model also involves a two-pronged approach to care termed the 'primary survey' and 'secondary survey'. In the primary survey, concentration is placed upon those factors which must be immediately addressed in order to keep the patient alive – diagnosing and treating injuries such as tension pneumothorax and cardiac tamponade, for example.

Trauma deaths have a tri-modal distribution, in other words, they happen at three different junctures:

- Immediate deaths occur at the scene and are due to non-survivable trauma such as massive head injury.
- Early deaths occur during the first 6 hours and may be due to evolving haemorrhage or similar preventable conditions.
- Late deaths occur days or weeks after trauma, and evolve from complications such as sepsis or multi-organ failure.

The primary survey seeks to identify and treat those preventable conditions causing early deaths in trauma patients.

Once the patient's immediately life-threatening conditions have been addressed, the secondary survey allows the trauma team more time to rigorously examine the patient for injuries from top to toe. This two-pronged approach ensures that the patient is effectively resuscitated, but also that minor injuries (a fractured thumb, for example) are not missed. The final stage, after the primary and secondary surveys are complete, is transfer of the stabilized patient to definitive care.

The ABCDE mnemonic explained in Chapter 2 (Box 2.10) provides a structured approach to trauma management. In practice, due to the nature of the trauma team approach, these stages happen rapidly and concurrently. In trauma training they are often taught and tested sequentially to ensure understanding of the individual components. The ABCDE model allows clinicians the rare luxury in medicine of a reductionist approach to a holistic problem.

Airway (with cervical spine control)

Management of the airway is of primary importance in trauma patients, since a patient with an obstructed airway will expire faster than one with impaired ventilation, and considerably before a patient with a haemorrhagic problem. Emphasis is placed concurrently on the management of the cervical spine, since immobilization of the neck is necessary to prevent or limit neurological damage until a potentially unstable spinal injury is ruled out. In all major trauma patients a spinal injury should be assumed until definitively excluded and spinal precautions must be maintained until this has been achieved.

Immobilization of the cervical spine is achieved in the trauma patient in one of two ways:

- A semi-rigid cervical collar, head blocks and tape
- Manual in-line immobilization.

Because spinal injury can occur anywhere in the spine it is necessary to immobilize the patient completely until an injury has been disproved (American College of Surgeons 2004).

If the patient attends the department without being immobilized, it will be necessary to 'strap and trap' him or her as soon as possible. If the patient is lying on a trolley, he or she should be approached from the front, and his or her head should be gently supported while an explanation is given of the necessity for spinal immobilization. This approach ensures that the patient does not have to turn his or her head towards you, which might happen if you approached from the side, or hyperextend his or her neck to see you if approached from the rear.

When manually immobilizing the patient, ensure you do not cover his or her ears. This is a common error, and makes your explanation very difficult! Sizing of the collar should be performed by someone familiar with the model in use in the department. There are adjustable models, as well as fixed sizes. Removal of jewellery is necessary before fitting the collar, and it is a good idea to check for any obvious wounds or bruising to the neck before covering it with the collar. Cervical collars for trauma use have open sections through which the trachea and neck veins can be observed, but it is a good idea to also check these important indicators of potential injury before fastening the collar.

Once the collar is secured, head blocks are applied to both sides of the patient's head, (to prevent it from rolling to either side), and tape is applied across the forehead and across the neckpiece of the collar (taking care not to obscure the view of the trachea and neck veins) (Figure 5.1). This tape is fastened to a rigid non-mobile surface on the trolley – it will afford little

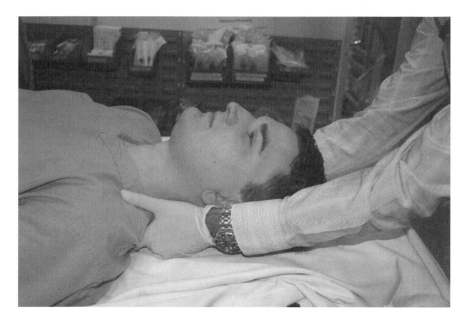

Figure 5.1   Spinal immobilization

support if it is applied to the cot-sides, and someone raises them to transfer the patient.

Once the patient is immobilized effectively with the three-point technique, manual immobilization can be released. There is one important caveat to this 'two method' rule in spinal immobilization. A patient who will not cooperate with spinal immobilization, either due of hypoxia, or the effects of drugs or alcohol, must not be forcibly immobilized. Strapping the patient down without his or her agreement will guarantee a combative patient whose potential spinal injury can only worsen because of the intervention. If the patient will tolerate manual immobilization, or even just a semi-rigid collar, then these should be used. Definitive immobilization may be achievable when the patient is calmer.

Another important caution is the patient with pre-existing spinal disease. If the patient has severe kyphosis, then attempting to 'straighten them out' in A&E will worsen any potential injury. Keeping the spine in the line which is normal for the patient will minimize any risk of deterioration.

As well as the collar, blocks and tape, patients are often transported to EDs on a transfer board (sometimes erroneously termed a 'spinal board'). These rigid boards are designed only for extrication and transfer of patients, and the patient should be removed from the board as soon as possible after arrival – at least at the end of the primary survey when the patient is log rolled. This will minimize the risks of pressure ulcer development and respiratory compromise associated with their long-term use.

A patient who vomits while immobilized presents a substantial risk of aspirating vomit into the airway. If the patient is still completely immobilized on the transfer board, this can be turned to 90 degrees by several people to enable the vomit to be expelled. If the patient is no longer on the board, or not fully strapped on, then the trolley should be tipped head down to 20 degrees, and the vomit suctioned from the patient's oropharynx. If the tip of the suction catheter proves too small to suction the vomit, the catheter should simply be removed from the tubing, and the tubing (which has a much wider bore) used.

In practice, spinal immobilization can be managed for extended periods with manual immobilization until the airway is assessed and secured. Trauma patients are at particular risk of airway obstruction, with potential injuries such as facial and mandibular trauma, laryngeal fracture, cricoid disruption, head injury and drug/alcohol ingestion, it is important to rigorously assess and regularly reassess the airway to ensure it remains patent, and to be able to respond rapidly and appropriately if airway support is required.

The simplest method of assessing the patient's airway is to speak to them. If they speak back, you know two things:

1   He or she is moving air past the vocal cords, and so the airway is (at least currently) intact.
2   Sufficient oxygen is getting to the brain so that he or she can make sense of what you are saying and formulate a response.

If the patient does not respond, or there are concerns about the airway, then it should be reassessed. The mouth should be opened so that it can be examined for foreign bodies, blood or vomit. Where these are discovered, they should be removed with suction or Magill forceps. Forceps should only be used if it is impossible to suction a foreign body, and then great care must be taken to ensure the material is not pushed further down the airway, with potentially catastrophic results. Well-fitting dentures should be left in place, as they help to maintain the integrity of the airway, loose dentures should be removed as a potential source of obstruction.

If the airway continues to show signs of obstruction (snoring, gurgling, stridor or abnormal breath sounds), a simple airway manoeuvre should be performed. A chin lift or jaw thrust manoeuvre can relieve obstruction by the tongue, which commonly falls back into the posterior oropharynx in unconscious patients.

After any intervention, it is important to reassess the patient – performing potentially life-saving manoeuvres is pointless unless you check to see if they have been effective. Remember, '*If you mess, reassess.*' If the airway

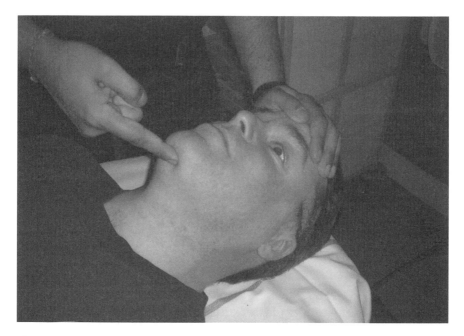

Figure 5.2 Head tilt, chin lift manoeuvre

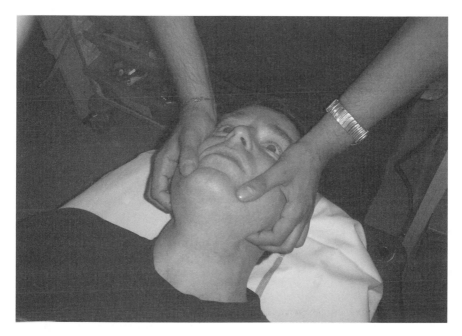

Figure 5.3 Jaw thrust manoeuvre

obstruction is relieved by the jaw thrust or chin lift, then a simple airway adjunct should be considered (unless you have someone who can perform the jaw thrust indefinitely). The two commonly available simple airway adjuncts are the oropharyngeal (or Guedel) and the nasopharyngeal airways (Chapter 9).

The oropharyngeal airway should be sized in accordance with the techniques outlined in Chapter 9. Once the airway has been placed, reassess the patient to ensure that it has had the desired effect. The oropharyngeal airway should be used as a temporizing measure until a definitive airway can be prepared, since a patient who is able to tolerate an oropharyngeal airway may have a level of consciousness associated with the need for intubation. In contrast, the nasopharyngeal airway is much better tolerated by conscious and semi-conscious patients, and is less likely to cause vomiting (American College of Surgeons 2004) (Chapter 9).

Head injury is often cited as a contraindication to the use of nasopharyngeal airways, but the only real contraindication to its use is in basal skull fracture. Guiding the airway parallel to the nasal floor rather than pointing it upwards, will reduce the risk of intracranial placement. Once the airway has been inserted, the patient should be reassessed.

If there is no improvement in the airway status after oropharyngeal or nasopharyngeal airway insertion, then the anaesthetist will consider advanced airway techniques.

Advanced airway techniques

Tracheal intubation is the gold standard in airway protection in trauma patients who cannot protect their own airway. Indications for intubation include a Glasgow coma scale of 8 or less (whatever the cause: a patient who has a GCS of 8 because of drugs or alcohol is as much at risk of airway obstruction as a patient with a head injury); inadequate ventilation; and injury to the upper airway.

Patients with inhalation or burn injury should be considered for elective intubation, even if they present with an apparently patent airway (Box 5.3). The rapid development of laryngeal oedema from exposure to extremely hot steam, gas or smoke may make intubation impossible once the airway starts to swell.

There are a number of reasons why intubation in the trauma patient is more difficult than, for example, elective surgery: there is less time to prepare and assess the patient's airway. There may be trauma to the airway itself, or facial trauma, which limits both the view and the passage of the tube. The patient must be kept immobilized, and so the optimal position for intubation may not be achieved. These factors may mean that the patient cannot be

Box 5.3 Indicators of inhalation injury

- Burns to the face or neck
- Singeing to eyebrows or nasal hair
- Carbon deposits and acute inflammatory changes in the oropharynx
- Carbonaceous sputum
- Hoarseness
- History of impaired mentation and/or confinement in a burning environment
- Explosion with burns to head and torso
- Carboxyhaemoglobin level > 10% if the patient has been involved in a fire (smokers may have a raised carboxyhaemoglobin).

(Adapted from American College of Surgeons 2004)

intubated, and if the anaesthetist is unable to pass an endotracheal tube, an alternative must be readily available.

Alternative airway management techniques

If the anaesthetist is unable to intubate the patient with an endotracheal tube, there are a variety of possible techniques to manage the airway.

The laryngeal mask airway (LMA) is a non-invasive and relatively simple product, which can often be inserted when endotracheal intubation is unsuccessful. It functions by occluding the oesophagus while ventilating the trachea. It does not provide protection against aspiration of stomach contents, however, and because it is inserted above the glottis, it cannot relieve laryngospasm or other subglottic problems. Despite these limitations, it is often the first line treatment for failed intubation in the trauma patient.

The intubating laryngeal mask airway is similar to the LMA, but allows an endotracheal tube to be passed through it for definitive intubation while still allowing ventilation.

If the anaesthetist is unable to ventilate the patient using the LMA, then more invasive methods must be considered. A patient with a critical loss of airway, who cannot be ventilated with a bag–valve–mask device, will require immediate intervention to prevent death.

A needle cricothyroidotomy involves placement of a large bore cannula (12–14 gauge) inserted through the cricothyroid membrane and into the trachea. The hub of the needle is then connected to an oxygen source, and the patient is ventilated with a Y connector or specialist insufflation device for a ratio of one second of oxygen delivery to four seconds without. It is a means of rapidly delivering oxygen to a patient with an obstructed airway, and is relatively safe. It is, however, a purely temporizing measure, since it does not allow effective gas exchange. This means that CO^2 accumulates, limiting the use of the technique to 30–45 minutes (American College of Surgeons 2004).

A surgical airway or cricothyroidotomy involves an incision through the cricothyroid membrane and the passage of an endotracheal or tracheostomy tube into the trachea. This allows effective ventilation, and is a relatively safe and secure airway. It is faster and easier to perform than a tracheostomy, and associated with few complications. Once the airway is secured through one of these methods, attention can turn to the patient's breathing.

Scenario 5.1   Head injury trauma

Paul is a 19-year-old man who is brought to the A&E department by ambulance. He has taken a large amount of alcohol and also four diazepam tablets in the last few hours. He was involved in a fight, during which he was knocked unconscious after being pushed down a flight of stairs. He has been aggressive, agitated and uncooperative with the ambulance staff, who have brought him in on a wheelchair.

His respiratory rate is 8, pulse 68 and blood pressure is 124/64. His GCS has yet to be formally evaluated, as the ambulance crew state he is refusing to answer their questions.

D *Data* (scientific facts): Paul has a history and signs (aggression, agitation) consistent with significant head injury. This has yet to be formally evaluated. He has recently consumed alcohol and diazepam and has yet to be spinally immobilized. His respiratory rate is low, but his pulse and blood pressure are normal.

E *Emotions* (intuition): Paul presents with a familiar pattern of injury post-assault on a background of alcohol and drug intoxication. This complicates his assessment and management, and has prevented the ambulance crew from immobilizing him or formally assessing his neurological status. An awareness of the potential for c-spine injury means he is placed in the resuscitation area and initially managed with manual immobilization until he is sufficiently calm to allow full immobilization.

Recognition of the potential for airway compromise related to his ingestion of alcohol and respiratory depressant medication, coupled with a head injury, means an early alert to the anaesthetist is necessary. The trauma team will already have been alerted, the patient having lost consciousness after a head injury.

A *Advantages*: clear explanation of all procedures is more likely to foster cooperation with Paul. His c-spine should be immobilized as much as he will allow. Early provision of oxygen through a non-rebreathe mask is necessary to support oxygenation where ventilation is reduced. Close attention to his respiratory rate and depth will demonstrate if assisted ventilation is needed – obtaining an arterial blood gas sample will inform the team if it is necessary.

Constant reassessment of Paul's airway is necessary, as well as initial assessment of his neurological status. It will be useful to have a baseline reading of his GCS as quickly as it can be obtained, so that any deterioration in his level of consciousness can be swiftly identified.

D *Disadvantages* (**differential diagnoses**): Paul's aggression and agitation may be a result of his head injury, his alcohol consumption or drug use, or a combination of all three. Hypoglycaemia should also be negated.

There is a risk of vomiting related to his alcohol use and head injury – there should be suction available, and someone constantly vigilant to tip his trolley and remove any vomit. An anti-emetic can be provided intravenously, but takes some time to work, and will not necessarily prevent vomiting.

If Paul's GCS declines to 8 or less, he should be intubated. Whether his respiratory and neurological compromise is caused by his head injury or by drugs and alcohol is not important – what is important is that his airway is protected.

Breathing (with ventilation)

After an obstructed airway, failed ventilation will swiftly claim the trauma victim unless the cause is promptly identified and managed. Every trauma patient should receive oxygen at 15 litres via a mask with a reservoir bag, even patients with a previous history of chronic obstructive pulmonary disease (Chapter 9).

Examination of the patient's breathing requires removal of his clothing. If his clothes have not already been removed, they should be taken off at this juncture.

Unfortunately it is often necessary to cut the patient's clothing, in order to remove them without mobilizing the spine. A pair of stout 'trauma scissors' can be purchased relatively cheaply, and will tackle the heaviest material. A stock of old (clean) clothing should be kept somewhere in the emergency department for those who may be discharged after having their clothing shredded.

Once the chest is fully exposed, it should be examined for the respiratory rate, any obvious injury or markings and any alteration in depth or rhythm of breathing on either side. A pulse oximeter should be applied, which will provide some information on the patient's respiratory status. It is not a reliable indicator of tissue oxygenation, however, and may give excellent readings in patients with carbon monoxide poisoning, who are in reality severely hypoxic. Measurement of arterial blood gasses is the gold standard evaluation of the effectiveness of ventilation, and should be undertaken if there is a suspicion of a traumatic thoracic injury.

A 'look, listen and feel' approach enables the team to assess and diagnose thoracic injuries effectively. Visual examination of the chest will reveal any obvious wounds or bruising. If the trachea and neck veins have not been previously examined, this should be done now. Palpation of the chest may elicit pain, crepitus and subcutaneous emphysema, while percussion of the chest will reveal hypo or hyper-resonance (a change in the percussion note relating to the presence of air or blood in the hemithorax). Auscultation of the chest with a stethoscope will reveal the presence or absence of breath sounds and enables the heart sounds to be assessed. These assessment techniques can reveal the signs of the major traumatic chest injuries recalled by the acronym ATOMFC:

Airway obstruction – Tension pneumothorax – Open pneumothorax – Massive haemothorax – Flail chest – Cardiac tamponade.

Airway obstruction

Major airway disruption may include tracheo-bronchial disruption from penetrating trauma to the neck and chest. The upper airway is well protected by the mandible and sternum, and by its natural elasticity. Blunt force trauma to the airway therefore most commonly arises from RTAs, where the patient is crushed or ejected from the vehicle with significant force. Injuries may present with few signs, and subcutaneous emphysema (the presence of air under the skin from a ruptured airway – often described as feeling like 'rice crispies' beneath the fingers) and a hoarse voice or stridor may be the only initial clues to a potentially disastrous clinical course.

These patients should be managed through the establishment of a patent airway, with appropriate imaging to establish the level and extent of injury (American College of Surgeons 2004).

Tension pneumothorax

The lungs are covered with a serous membrane called the visceral pleura. A corresponding layer, the parietal pleura, lines the surface of the chest wall, the upper surface of the diaphragm and the mediastinum. Normally these surfaces stick closely together, so that the pleural cavity (the space between the two layers) is very small. A pneumothorax arises from a breach in the visceral, parietal or mediastinal pleura, allowing the passage of air into the pleural cavity. This increases the distance between the visceral and parietal layers.

A 'simple' pneumothorax is such a pocket of air, and may be drained, either with a needle or a chest tube. If it is small enough, the patient may be sent home the same day with advice to return if dyspnoea occurs. Sometimes, however, the breach in the pleura develops a 'one-way valve' effect, where air can escape into the pleural cavity on inspiration, but is prevented from returning on expiration by a clot or other tissue. This is a 'tension' pneumothorax, and is a common manifestation in traumatic injury. It may arise from penetrating injury to the lung parenchyma, a tear in the lung from deceleration injury, or rupture from crush injury. Continued accumulation of air in the pleural cavity increases the pressure within the affected hemithorax, eventually collapsing the lung, pushing the mediastinum and collapsed lung towards the other side of the chest. The pressure on the great vessels may eventually compromise venous return, and if the pressure continues, cardiac arrest may occur.

Fortunately these physiological effects leave substantial clues for the alert practitioner. A patient with a tension pneumothorax will develop dyspnoea as the lung surface available for gas exchange reduces. In order to compensate, the patient will become tachypnoeic, and as hypoxia sets in, he or she will become increasingly agitated. Objective signs arise from the collapse of the lung – there will be a progressive decrease in breath sounds, and a 'hyperresonance' to percussion on the affected side. As the lung collapses, the thoracic cavity is filled with air rather than lung tissue, and consequently the percussion note is more 'drum-like', or hyperresonant. This is in contrast to the hyporesonance, or dullness, encountered when the thorax is filled with blood in a haemothorax.

Other signs, which may be present, are tracheal deviation, due to massive mediastinal shift in the opposite direction to the pressure (so, in a right-sided tension pneumothorax, the trachea may be deviated to the left side), and distended neck veins from venous obstruction. These signs may not be present, however – tracheal deviation is a very late sign and easily missed, and distension of neck veins may not occur in a patient with hypovolaemia (Leigh-Smith and Harris 2005).

Prompt treatment is required to relieve the intrathoracic tension and restore the negative pressure needed to allow lung expansion. The definitive treatment is a tube thoracostomy (a tube inserted through the chest wall to allow drainage of the air in the pleural cavity). This takes time to set up and perform, however, during which the patient's condition may become critical. The pressure can be immediately relieved, however, by the placement of a large bore cannula through the second intercostal space at the mid-clavicular line on the affected side. This is called a needle thoracocentesis, and is both a therapeutic and diagnostic manoeuvre – a hiss of escaping air is supposed to be

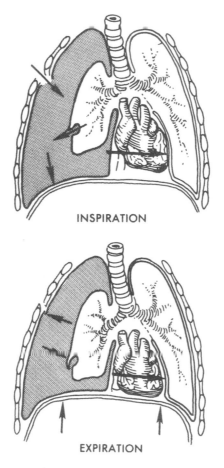

INSPIRATION

EXPIRATION

Figure 5.4 Tension pneumothorax

audible in a positive thoracocentesis, as the air in the lungs escapes under tension through the cannula. In practice this may not be easy to hear in a noisy trauma room with oxygen being delivered at 15 litres close to the site. Reliance should not be placed on a positive or negative 'hiss of air', but rather on clinical suspicion and reassessment after the procedure. Reassessment should demonstrate improved air entry, a normal or less resonant percussion note and a marked improvement in dyspnoea. A definitive chest tube should be inserted as soon as possible. Until it is inserted, the cannula should be left in place and open to the air, so that the lung does not re-tension.

Open pneumothorax

Penetrating trauma to the chest wall may result in a 'sucking chest wound', where air enters the wound on inspiration, allowing the intrathoracic and atmospheric pressures to equalize. This causes ineffective ventilation, and if the wound is larger than two-thirds of the size of the patient's trachea, then air will enter the wound rather than the trachea – further impairing oxygenation. The patient will present with a thoracic wound, which may demonstrate the characteristic 'sucking sound' as air enters the thorax. There will be signs of hypoxia and chest pain.

Treatment requires the placement of a sterile occlusive dressing, which is taped on three sides to create a one-way valve. This allows air to escape from the chest on expiration but not to re-enter it on inspiration, as the dressing is sucked onto the surface of the chest. A gloved hand can be used as a temporizing measure until a dressing is prepared – occluding the wound on inspiration, and removing the hand on expiration. This should be followed by placement of a tube thoracostomy before surgical exploration and closure of the wound.

Massive haemothorax

A haemothorax (blood in the pleural cavity) may arise from both blunt and penetrating thoracic trauma. Laceration of the pulmonary parenchyma, intercostal arteries and major bronchial vessels can cause occult bleeding – each hemithorax being capable of holding 50 per cent of the patient's circulating volume. A small amount of bleeding may be well tolerated, but larger amounts will cause tachycardia and hypotension in response to hypovolaemia (neck veins may be flat as a result), dyspnoea, reduced breath sounds as the lung is displaced by blood, and a consequent hyporesonant percussion note.

Treatment involves fluid replacement, surgical referral and tube thoracostomy to evacuate the blood and re-expand the lung. If there is an initial drainage of 1500mls or more, or continued drainage of 200mls per hour for two hours or more, then patients should be considered for surgical intervention to control the bleeding (American College of Surgeons 2004).

The chest tube should ideally be placed at the base of the thorax for optimal fluid drainage, and should be a large bore (28–30 minimum – Laws et al. 2003). Once the chest tube has been inserted, the patient should be re-assessed – dyspnoea should improve, but hypotension and tachycardia may remain due to continued hypovolaemia.

Flail chest

A flail chest occurs when two or more ribs are fractured in two or more places, or when the ribs are detached from the sternum. Associated with significant blunt force trauma, flail chest indicates the potential for substantial pulmonary contusion. Diagnosis is through recognition of the 'paradoxical movement' of the flail segment. As the patient breathes in, the segment (which is no longer attached to the thoracic wall) 'caves in' as pressure within the pleural space decreases. Expiration makes the segment 'swell up' as the pleural pressure increases. Palpation of bony crepitus will aid diagnosis.

Arterial blood gasses should be monitored to establish the degree of underlying lung contusion. Patients with significantly impaired gas exchange should be considered for elective ventilation, although most patients can be managed with analgesia and oxygen. The extent of the flail segment itself is not as important as the underlying contusion. The importance of a flail chest may lie in highlighting the significant force involved in the incident, with odds of death being significantly higher in patients with multiple rib fractures.

Cardiac tamponade

The heart is encased in a fibrous layer called the pericardium. The pericardium has two layers, the visceral layer covers the heart's surface, and the parietal layer surrounds it. The pericardial space between the two layers normally contains a small amount of fluid (less than 50 mls) to lubricate the beating heart. If the heart is damaged (normally from penetrating trauma) and bleeds into the pericardial space, the stiff parietal layer will not stretch to accommodate the additional fluid. In other conditions where fluid also accumulates, such as pericarditis, the pericardium may gradually stretch to accommodate up to two litres before cardiac compression occurs (Hawley et al. 2003).

In acute traumatic injury, the accumulation of only 50–100mls of blood may increase the intrapericardial pressure to such an extent that diastolic filling and venous return are severely compromised. Signs of shock (in this case, cardiogenic) will become apparent as the pressure in the pericardial space rises to meet the pressure within the heart itself. Pericardial tamponade should therefore always be considered in a patient with penetrating trauma where the degree of shock is inconsistent with apparent injury

Signs of pericardial tamponade include 'Beck's Triad', consisting of hypotension, muffled heart sounds (as contraction is reduced by pressure, and sound is insulated by additional fluid), and distended neck veins (from elevated venous pressure). These signs may not always be apparent, however. With the presence of hypovolaemic shock the neck veins may remain flat, and heart sounds may be difficult to evaluate in an obese patient in a noisy resuscitation room. A high index of suspicion should be maintained in a patient with penetrating thoraco-abdominal injury, with measurement of the pulse pressure at 5-minute intervals to reveal the beginning of the shock state (Chapter 2).

There are several treatment options for the relief of pericardial tamponade. A thoracostomy, where the chest is opened sufficiently to visualize and manipulate the heart, is the optimal procedure in the hands of a skilled practitioner. This is because the blood in the pericardial space is often clotted, and cannot be removed by means of a needle as in pericardiocentesis.

The 'pericardial window' procedure is a surgical technique, which entails an incision below the sternum to enable direct visualization of the pericardium. This is followed by cutting a small opening in the pericardium to evacuate a clot or fluid from the pericardial space if this is seen. Although it is less invasive than thoracotomy, both of these procedures are best performed in theatre by a surgeon experienced in the technique under a general anaesthetic.

In practice, with a patient in extremis and a likely diagnosis of pericardial tamponade (history of penetrating thoracic trauma, shock in the absence of obvious haemorrhage), a needle pericardiocentesis is the procedure of choice.

A pericardiocentesis can be rapidly performed with minimal equipment in the resuscitation room. If ultrasound is available, it may be rapidly used to demonstrate the presence of haemopericardium, confirming the diagnosis. A 6-inch, 16 to 18 gauge over-the-needle catheter is attached to a 50 ml syringe with a three-way tap and advanced through the skin just below the sternum towards the heart. While this is being done, the cardiac monitor must be observed for signs of an injury pattern (ST segment elevation, ectopic activity). This demonstrates that the needle has been advanced too far, and is penetrating the ventricular myocardium. If this occurs, the needle is withdrawn until the tracing returns to normal. In departments where echocardiography is available, this can also be used to safely guide the catheter tip into the pericardial space.

Once blood begins to be aspirated from the pericardium, attention should remain on the ECG tracing, since the myocardium will approach the edge of the pericardium as the fluid in the pericardial space decreases (American College of Surgeons 2004). As much blood as possible should be aspirated, and the catheter should then be secured in place for re-aspiration if required. The patient should be rapidly transferred for definitive specialist surgical intervention after reassessment.

Once any major thoracic injuries have been identified and managed, attention can move to assessment of the patient's circulatory status.

Circulation (with haemorrhage control)

Patients presenting in shock with a history of trauma are assumed to be hypovolaemic from haemorrhage until proven otherwise. Obvious heavily bleeding wounds can be managed by direct pressure immediately the patient arrives, but should not divert the team from dealing with the airway and breathing. A patient can lose blood from a variety of places, characterized by the phrase, 'on the floor and four more'. 'On the floor' refers to blood loss at scene, which should be ascertained from the paramedics or any witnesses to the incident.

The 'four more' places a patient can bleed from (and without immediately obvious external sign) are:

- chest
- abdomen
- pelvis
- long bones.

The abdomen can be further subdivided into the peritoneal and retroperitoneal spaces, which are separate from each other. The peritoneal cavity contains the liver and spleen, both highly vascular organs, as well as the stomach and gall bladder. The retroperitoneal space contains the kidneys and ureters, the pancreas and significant vasculature, including the abdominal aorta and inferior vena cava. This is significant, because tests applied to the peritoneal cavity, such as diagnostic peritoneal lavage (DPL – see below) do not reveal injury to structures in the retroperitoneum.

The first act in the circulation phase of trauma treatment is assessment. You cannot reassess your patient unless you have a baseline from which to do so. A pulse should be taken manually (not read from the monitor). This is important for two reasons:

1 The monitor does not allow you to judge the character of the pulse – is it weak/thready?
2 The presence or absence of a pulse at particular locations can tell you roughly what the patient's blood pressure is. A palpable radial pulse indicates a systolic blood pressure of around 80–90mmHg, a femoral pulse 70mmHg and a carotid pulse indicates 60mmHg.

A blood pressure measurement should also be performed, being careful to record the pulse pressure (the difference between the systolic and diastolic pressure) as a separate entry. It is useful to do this in a separate colour pen, as it can become confused with the pulse on the chart. This figure will reduce (as the patient begins to compensate through vasoconstriction, the diastolic figure will rise, while the systolic remains constant) before the blood pressure starts to fall. This, along with tachypnoea, tachycardia and agitation, are the earliest signs of shock.

As compensatory mechanisms are activated, peripheral vasoconstriction drives much-needed oxygenated blood to the central circulation, leaving the peripheries pale and cool – another relatively early sign of shock. This is another reason to keep your patient covered once he or she has been assessed for injury – removing someone's clothes in a relatively cold resuscitation room will make their skin cool at the best of times.

The patient should also be placed on a cardiac monitor at this stage, and the rhythm noted. If there is an arrhythmia, then an ECG reading should be obtained at an early juncture.

Fluid resuscitation

Two large bore cannulae (size 16 or larger) should be inserted one in each arm in the forearm or antecubital veins. Blood should be obtained and sent for blood type and cross-matching, as well as relevant laboratory studies. Traditionally once access is obtained one or two litres of warmed Hartmann's solution is infused as rapidly as possible. Hartmann's is used rather than normal saline because its metabolism in the liver and kidneys generates bicarbonate, which may buffer the lactic acid generated in shock (remember that as cells begin to respire anaerobically, lactic acid is produced). Large volumes of normal saline, on the other hand, may cause a hyperchloraemic acidosis, and should be avoided except in hypochloraemic and alkalotic patients.

The fluid should be warmed to 39 degrees by passage through a fluid warmer (or by storage in a specially controlled warming cupboard) to prevent potentially catastrophic coagulopathy and hypothermia associated with the transfusion of large amounts of cold fluids in trauma resuscitation (Kauver and Wade 2005).

A large amount has been written on the subject of the 'colloid versus crystalloid' debate over many years. Colloids are composed of large protein and sugar molecules that remain in the intravascular space, as they are so large they cannot cross the capillary wall or cell membrane. They increase the osmotic pressure and 'draw fluid in', thus effectively maintaining blood pressure. Crystalloids are composed of much smaller solutes, and also hydrate the extra-cellular spaces. Since our cellular environment reflects the 'primordial sea' from which life evolved, the maintenance of fluid and sodium in the extracellular environment is (at least initially) desirable.

Large-scale studies of crystalloid and colloid use have been unable to demonstrate a definitive benefit for either solution in trauma patients.

Crystalloids, because they diffuse into the interstitial and intracellular spaces, must be given at a ratio of 3 litres to each litre of blood lost. Colloids can be given at an equal volume to blood loss, since they remain in the intravascular space. The cost of colloids is so great, however (colloid is around 11 times the cost of crystalloid), that they are not used, since research demonstrates that crystalloids replace intravascular loss with equivalent mortality at a much lower outlay. The ATLS faculty recommend titrating the amount of fluid against the degree of shock and the patient's response to the initial fluid challenge (American College of Surgeons 2004). The degree of shock is estimated from a set of parameters including the pulse rate and blood pressure, respiratory rate and urine output (Table 5.1)

The average human has approximately 70mls/kg of blood volume: in a 70kg person this is 4.9 litres. Death is assured after the loss of approximately 50 per cent of circulating volume, and hypotension only occurs after the loss of approximately 30 per cent of the blood volume. Plainly then, to wait for a drop in blood pressure before intervening with fluid replacement would be criminally negligent. As can be seen from Table 5.1, before this happens there

Table 5.1 Degrees of shock

	CLASS 1	CLASS 2	CLASS 3	CLASS 4
Blood loss (ml)	Up to 750	750–1500	1500–2000	>2000
Pulse rate	⇑	⇑	⇑⇑	⇑⇑⇑
Blood pressure	⟺	⟺	⇓⇓	⇓⇓⇓
Pulse pressure (MmHg)	⟺	⇓	⇓	⇓
Respiratory rate	⟺	⇑	⇑⇑	⇑⇑⇑
Urine output (ml/hr)	⟺	⇓	⇓⇓	⇓⇓⇓

Notes: ⟺ Normal; ⬆ Raised; ⬇ Decreased;

⬆ Mild; ⬆⬆ Moderate; ⬆⬆⬆ Severe.

Source: Adapted from American College of Surgeons (2004)

are significant clues in increased pulse and respiratory rates, a narrowing pulse pressure and decreased urine output. It is against these parameters that fluid resuscitation is measured.

There has been extensive discussion around the concept of 'permissive hypotension' in trauma patients. This approach consists of maintaining the blood pressure at a level below normal, but sufficient to perfuse the major organs (Chapter 2), until the source of haemorrhage can be identified and repaired in theatre. If a radial pulse can be felt, the blood pressure is considered sufficient. The radial pulse and thus, organ perfusion are maintained by infusing increments of 250mls avoiding a sudden increase in systolic pressure. The rationale for this is that left alone a vascular injury may clot, preventing further bleeding. Large volume fluid resuscitation may dilute clotting factors and may mechanically destroy evolving clots through increased pressure 'popping the clot'. This approach is extensively used by military trauma teams (Krausz 2006).

Animal trials have demonstrated some benefit from limiting initial fluid replacement in traumatic injuries. There are also persuasive arguments for limiting fluid resuscitation in patients with injuries which are not readily accessible for surgical repair, such as posterior pelvic injuries. Unfortunately there is very little evidence to support the use of either large volume resuscitation or permissive hypotension (Kwann et al. 2003). Perhaps the best approach is for treatment to be based on the experience and judgement of the clinician, with attention to the individual presentation before them. Close attention to the signs of shock can aid the team in monitoring the patient's response to haemorrhage and fluid replacement, and is a vital nursing role.

Once fluids have been infused, then the patient should be reassessed to establish their effect. Further fluid replacement decisions can then be made, informed by the patient's haemodynamic response. Remember that individual patient factors can confound your expectations of 'normal' haemodynamic reactions, particularly in the groups in Box 5.4. Examination of the patient for sites of potential haemorrhage is then undertaken.

The chest

The chest will have already been fully examined as part of the breathing assessment, but can be reassessed at any time. There should be awareness that both cardiac tamponade and tension pneumothorax can cause shock in the absence of significant haemorrhage. Fractures of the first three ribs should prompt close examination and frequent reassessment of the patient – they indicate a very high impact injury, as these ribs are well protected by the shoulder girdles and associated musculature.

Box 5.4 Confounding haemodynamic factors

The old:	Reduced cardiac compliance and a decreased sympathetic response may mean elderly patients do not respond as well as younger patients.
The cold:	Hypothermic patients are already significantly vasoconstricted. Coagulopathy is more likely in a hypothermic patient, so rapid re-warming should occur (while monitoring the blood pressure – a sudden increase in the size of the vascular bed through warm vasodilation may cause significant hypotension).
Going for gold:	The extremely fit athlete may have an enormous cardiac output, and a normal resting heart rate of 40. A rate of 75 in these patients reveals a significant tachycardia.
Adding to the fold:	Pregnant patients have altered anatomy and physiology, with increased heart rate, and decreased blood pressure. Foetal monitoring should be undertaken, and the gravid uterus should be manually displaced to the left to prevent compression of the inferior vena cava (the use of a Cardiff wedge is contraindicated in suspected spinal injury).
BP controlled:	Drugs such as beta-blockers can maintain a relative bradycardia in the face of significant shock. Beware also the patient with a constant heart rate of 70 – check for a pacemaker!

The abdomen

The abdomen can be examined in four quadrants (left upper, left lower, right upper, right lower) to establish pain, distension, guarding, and any obvious external signs of potential injury (e.g., severe bruising over the spleen, a wound over the liver) (Chapter 7). In penetrating injury from knives or guns it is important to establish the type of weapon involved. Knives can vary in length from a few centimetres to a metre – a weapon large enough to reach any part of the body. If possible, the examination can be guided to a certain extent by knowledge of the mechanism of injury – was the patient stabbed? If so, how many times and with what kind of weapon? Has it been recovered so it can be viewed? Questions about the type of gun used in a shooting are particularly important. A bullet from a low calibre pistol enters a patient with considerably lower energy than a rifle bullet. Bullets begin to 'somersault' as they hit tissue and bone, causing massive destruction associated with enormous energy transfer (Dickinson 2004).

Practitioners should be aware that a bullet or knife wound may track a considerable distance from its entry point. A bullet entering the abdomen may lodge in the cervical spine, while a knife wound to the chest may cause abdominal injury. An entry wound may give some clue to underlying damage, but it cannot reveal the extent and seriousness of tissue destruction.

Blunt trauma spreads its damage over a wider area, and is much more common in the UK, arising from RTAs and falls. Injury results from direct transfer of deceleration forces to the body, where organs have different deceleration rates than surrounding tissue. This may cause the liver and other highly vascular organs to tear loose from their blood supply, causing catastrophic haemorrhage.

History is once again extremely important to establish the forces involved, and gain some clues to potential injury. If a patient is involved in a RTA, it is important to know the speeds involved. A car crashing into a wall at 15mph will not generate enormous force. A two-car collision with both cars travelling at 40mph adds up to an equivalent force of 80mph, however, and is considerably more likely to generate serious injuries.

Asking about damage to the cars involved will give important clues, if speed cannot be accurately recalled. A car, which has been 'written off' at scene, will have sustained much higher energy transfer than a car with a small dent in the boot. It is also important to know whether the patient was wearing their seatbelt, where in the car they were in relation to the forces involved, and whether they broke the windscreen with their head. All of these questions can give important clues to injury. We know that some injuries are more likely in RTAs (femoral and pelvic fractures, for example, from force transmitted by the dashboard through the seated patient's legs), but still require diagnostic aids to help us establish organ injury.

Fortunately there are several aids to diagnosis of underlying injury in the trauma patient.

Diagnostic peritoneal lavage

Diagnostic peritoneal lavage (DPL) is an invasive procedure, which involves passing a catheter into the abdominal cavity and infusing fluid through it. Draining the fluid back out reveals the presence of frank bleeding, bile or faecal or food materials, which demonstrate the presence of intra-abdominal injury. It is a sensitive and specific test for abdominal injury, which is relatively simple to perform in the resuscitation room. Unfortunately, not many surgeons in the UK are experienced in the technique. Even if it can be performed, there are not many haematology departments capable of analysing the fluid and providing the result in a timely fashion.

DPL cannot be repeated, and subsequent computed tomography (CT) or ultrasound examinations are compromised by fluid, which invariably remains in the abdomen after lavage. For these reasons, coupled with the fact that DPL does not reveal retroperitoneal injury, it has been overtaken by ultrasound and

CT as the examination of choice for patients with traumatic abdominal injury (Jansen and Logie 2005).

Focused abdominal sonography for trauma

Focused abdominal sonography for trauma (FAST) involves rapid evaluation of injury with ultrasound. With experienced operators it is highly sensitive and specific, and can be used to examine the chest and pelvis as well as the abdomen. It is fast, non-invasive, repeatable and does not interfere with subsequent CT examination. Unlike DPL, FAST does not require the patient to have a urinary catheter and nasogastric tube (to decompress the stomach and bladder in order to minimize risk of injury). If a skilled operator is available, FAST is an excellent method of quickly evaluating traumatic injury in the resuscitation area (Ollerton et al. 2006). FAST may need to be followed by CT, however, in order to pinpoint specific injury, and to rule out abdominal injury in patients with a negative FAST result, but for whom clinical suspicion persists.

Computed tomography

Computed tomography (CT) can be rapidly performed once the patient is in the scanner, and provides extraordinary detail of specific injury. It is particularly useful in examination for retroperitoneal injury, where FAST is not as accurate and DPL is valueless. There are problems with CT in the trauma patient, however. It can only be used in cooperative patients, since they must lie still in the scanner.

Haemodynamically compromised patients are placed at additional risk by being removed from the resuscitation room to the scanner; and large doses of radiation are necessary to derive the complex images, which give CT its value.

The pelvis and long bones

The pelvis can hide a very large volume of blood with no external evidence. It has large vascular vessels running through it, and fracture of the pelvis is associated with enormous force, (the pelvis being a series of rings – an extremely stable and strong structure). The pelvis can be examined by looking for signs of direct injury (bruising, perineal or scrotal haematoma, crepitus and pain). The pelvis should not be 'sprung', however (a method of examination which involves pushing down on the iliac crests to establish whether they move, due to fracture or dislocation). This examination may worsen vascular injury, and is not necessary – a pelvic X-ray can be obtained as part of the 'trauma series' of chest, cervical spine and pelvis. Unstable pelvic fractures can be 'wrapped' in a sheet to stabilize them prior to definitive splintage – there are also various kinds of belt available for pelvic stabilization, but a sheet tied around the patient serves the purpose.

Fractures of the femur can cause significant blood loss (up to a litre, and more in open fracture). Visibly exsanguinating wounds can be controlled initially with direct pressure, but for femoral fracture, splintage should be instituted as soon as possible. This will help reduce pain, and may prevent catastrophic haemorrhage in a patient with bilateral fractures – the application of a splint can be life-saving, therefore, and should not be long delayed. Checking the patient's distal pulses before and after applying a traction splint will ensure you have not worsened the patient's condition.

Burns

Fluid loss from burns can be catastrophic, and must be replaced rapidly and accurately. An assessment of the size of a burn must be made using the rule of nines (where each anatomic region represents 9 per cent of the body surface area). Crystalloids are then given using the formula 4mls/kg multiplied by the percentage of burned tissue (superficial burns, i.e., simple erythema or 'sunburn' are ignored). For a 50kg patient with 20 per cent burns, the fluid requirement would be 4×50×20, which is 4000mls. One half of this must be given in the first eight hours post-burn injury: if the patient was burned two hours before fluids start, they must be given in six hours. The remaining half will be given over 16 hours (American College of Surgeons 2004).

Once the patient's circulation has been stabilized, attention can turn to potential head injury, notated under the ABC model as D for 'Disability'.

Scenario 5.2   Road traffic accident trauma
Freda is a 34-year-old teacher. She is a cross-Channel swimming record holder, having recently swum the English Channel in the fastest time ever for a woman. On one of her daily training runs, she has been forced off the pavement and into the path of a lorry, which has run over the lower half of her body.   She complains of significant pain in both her legs, and refuses to wear a cervical collar, stating her neck is not painful. Her observations at scene were respiratory rate 24, Pulse 94, Blood pressure 115/98, and GCS 15/15.

D *Data* (scientific facts): Freda has a mechanism of injury associated with significant blunt force trauma to the lower body. Her systolic blood pressure and pulse are normal, and her respiratory rate is high. In the light of her extraordinary fitness, however, her haemodynamic status is more sinister. When you learn that her normal resting pulse rate is 42, it becomes plain that she is significantly tachycardic.

Examination of the diastolic blood pressure reveals a compensatory rise, which has narrowed the pulse pressure to 17 – a low figure suggesting approaching maximum compensation.

E *Emotions* (intuition): Freda has been subjected to enormous force and a full trauma team approach is required. Provision of oxygen is necessary to maximize oxygenation of her remaining blood volume. Spinal immobilization should be undertaken, despite her insistence that she has no neck pain. She has a major distracting injury, which may mask the pain from a spinal injury. A full assessment of her airway and breathing status will be undertaken before her circulatory assessment.

Instinct tells you that Freda is at very high risk for significant haemorrhage from blunt force trauma to her legs, pelvis and possibly her abdomen as well. Two large bore cannulae should be inserted and fluid titrated to maintain organ perfusion. Baseline recordings of both pulse and blood pressure will guide further resuscitation. An estimate of Freda's blood loss can be gained by her response to this initial fluid challenge.

A *Advantages*: swiftly removing Freda's clothing enables a rapid assessment of any obvious external wounds, and a visual check for femoral deformity or bruising. An awareness of the severity of the mechanism of injury should prompt a request for cross-matched blood, and also for immediate supply of O negative blood for rapid replacement of oxygen-carrying capacity. Pain relief should be given rapidly to relieve the significant pain in her legs. Splinting of her femoral fractures should be undertaken early to minimize continuing blood loss and pain.

D *Disadvantages* (differential diagnoses): Freda requires rapid assessment and management of a serious injury. Concentrating solely on her femoral fractures may miss occult abdominal and pelvic injury. Use of a FAST scan may enable a rapid rule in/out for other injuries. She cannot be transferred to CT for evaluation as she is extremely haemodynamically unstable. There should be early transfer to theatre for operative intervention for any pelvic fracture, and a high index of suspicion for concomitant abdominal injury.

Disability

The primary insult in traumatic head injury has already occurred at scene. The job of the trauma team is to minimize secondary injury from hypoxia and hypotension (Chapter 8). Patients with a GCS of 8 or less are literally comatose – close attention must be paid to the airway until the GCS either rapidly improves or the patient is intubated. If the patient is to be sedated or paralysed, it is vital to obtain measurement of the GCS and pupillary reaction, as knowledge of the patient's clinical condition will guide subsequent treatment (American College of Surgeons 2004). In most units, the patient will be stabilized and transferred to the nearest neurosurgical provider after CT. Before that is done, the primary survey must be completed, and this requires the patient to be fully exposed.

Exposure/environmental control

So far, we have seen only a maximum of two-thirds of our patient – we have not seen any of her back. In order to fully assess the patient they must be 'log rolled' (the spine is maintained in immobilization, as it must be examined for tenderness before it can be 'cleared'). A log roll procedure requires six people; the inclusion of the patient is vital to the success of the procedure. A full explanation of what you are about to do will hopefully guarantee cooperation and a smooth process in a conscious patient.

The person in charge of the log roll is the person at the patient's head – normally the anaesthetist. They are responsible for ensuring that c-spine immobilization is maintained and that the airway is protected (if necessary) during the procedure. Three others are ranged down the length of the patient, with their hands in the positions seen in Figure 5.5. The tallest is at the patient's shoulders, the shortest at the feet. The examining doctor explains the procedure to the patient – particularly remembering to tell the patient if they are going to do a PR examination (a finger is placed in the patient's rectum to check for muscular tone, which may be absent in spinal injury). All too often this is not explained, and then only in a very rudimentary fashion, when the patient is already rolled onto his or her side.

Before the log roll takes place, the leader ensures the brakes on the trolley are on, announces the words he or she will use for the turn (normally '1, 2, 3, turn') and advises the patient to remain still throughout the procedure. The patient can then be turned through 90 degrees and his or her back examined while spinal immobilization is maintained. The entire spinal column must be examined, from the occipital cervical junction to the sacrum, and the presence of any pain or swelling, bruising or misalignment noted (Harris and Sethi 2006).

The patient must be kept warm throughout her stay. Hypothermia will worsen the patient's condition, and must be avoided, despite the need to assess and reassess the patient regularly in a cold resuscitation room. Use of warm air blanket systems is suitable, and fluids are, of course warmed to 39 degrees. Use of foil blankets on a cool patient is *not* suitable – if we want to

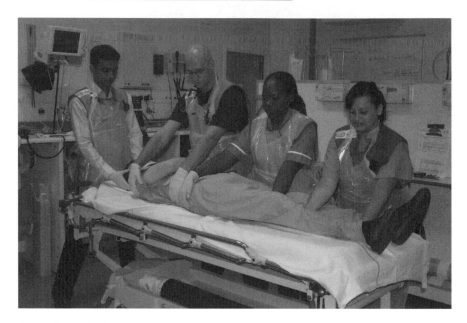

Figure 5.5 The log roll

keep someone cold, then wrapping them in insulating foil is a good way to do it.

Once the primary survey has been completed, the secondary survey can begin. This may occur some time later, after the patient has been to theatre. It involves a complete head-to-toe examination and further history taking. If you have managed to deliver your patient to the secondary survey with life and limb intact, you have completed you task as a trauma practitioner.

Conclusion

Trauma is an interesting and dynamic subject – practitioners who are interested in expanding their knowledge are advised to go to www.trauma.org, where they will find excellent resources for multi-disciplinary trauma care.

6 Gynaecological and obstetric emergencies

Michelle Stanton

Introduction

Gynaecological and obstetric emergencies are a frequent reason for both a patient's attendance and subsequent admission. The aim of this chapter is to explore some of these common presentations and highlight areas where clinicians who have a foundation of relevant knowledge and understanding can dramatically influence the care received by the patient.

Bleeding in early and late pregnancy

Bleeding in early and late pregnancy is among the commonest of gynaeco-logical and obstetric presentations to the ED, bleeding in early pregnancy can be due to a number of causes as listed in Box 6.1.

Box 6.1   Causes of bleeding in early pregnancy
• Threatened miscarriage • Inevitable miscarriage • Incomplete miscarriage • Complete miscarriage • Missed miscarriage • Ectopic pregnancy • Gestational trophoblastic disease – molar pregnancy • Local causes such as infection, polyps, cervical ectopy.

The main symptoms are:

• Bleeding: spotting of blood or haemorrhage

- Pain
- The passage of tissue: the products of conception (POC).

Bleeding, regardless of the stage of the pregnancy, should never be under-estimated as it can suddenly develop into a life-threatening haemorrhage, particularly if it is due to an ectopic pregnancy.

Miscarriage is the spontaneous expulsion of the products of conception (POC) prior to the 24th week of pregnancy; it is most common in the first trimester. Miscarriage can present in a number of ways and is classified accordingly (see Box 6.2).

Box 6.2   Classification of miscarriage
• Threatened miscarriage • Inevitable miscarriage • Incomplete miscarriage • Complete miscarriage • Missed miscarriage • Recurrent or habitual miscarriage • Septic miscarriage

Scenario 6.1   Miscarriage

Jane is a 26-year-old primigravida; last menstrual period (LMP) was ten weeks ago. She presents with a 2-day history of spotting, which is becoming heavier, and cramp-like pains. Jane has a respiratory rate of 14, a regular radial pulse rate of 92 bpm and a blood pressure of 120/72 mmHg. Her temperature is 36.7°C. Jane is very anxious.

D *Data* (**scientific facts**): the clinical history is suggestive of a threatened miscarriage. Threatened miscarriage will commonly present with slight to mild vaginal spotting/bleeding, pain is not always present and is commonly described as 'cramp-like' pains and/or backache. The severity of pain should, nonetheless, be carefully assessed and monitored.

While Jane appears to be haemodynamically stable, a sudden PV haemorrhage can be haemodynamically devastating, therefore, women presenting with any amount of vaginal bleeding must be taken very seriously and clinically prioritized on their actual and potential problems. The initial management should focus on the airway, breathing and circulation (RCUK 2006).

E *Emotions* (**intuition**): experienced clinicians recognize that Jane's presentation has the potential to become life-threatening.

Jane will be cared for in an area where facilities are freely available in case of sudden compromise. Due to Jane's distress, her privacy must be respected.

A *Advantages*: prompt diagnosis and treatment can reduce maternal mortality. Ectopic pregnancy must be excluded. Vaginal bleeding in early pregnancy can range from mild to life-threatening haemorrhage and in some cases predispose toward maternal death. Early specialist referral is essential; in the meantime an experienced emergency physician may be able to complement the nurse in the initial assessment.

Many emergency departments will have a fast track system for presentations related to PV bleeding in order that patients are cared for in a more suitable environment. In the meantime Jane should be subject to regular observations; these will comprise pulse, blood pressure, respiratory rate and pulse oximetry recordings every 15–30 minutes dependent on clinical condition. A large bore venous cannula should be inserted, with cross-match/group and save a priority, routine bloods will also be requested, in addition, an antibody screen to check Rhesus status and a clotting screen may be necessary. Intravenous fluids will be infused titrated to her needs.

Monitoring of vaginal loss must also take place with pads being saved to examine what has been passed and an estimate made of the amount of bleeding. A pregnancy test whereby beta-HCG is measured is useful in confirming diagnosis of pregnancy, an ultrasound scan should be performed as soon as possible. This is now the most effective investigation to aid diagnosis as the type of miscarriage can be diagnosed and, importantly, whether the foetus is viable. Visualization of the foetal heart by ultrasound scanning differentiates between a woman with a viable pregnancy, who can be discharged, and a woman with a non-viable or ectopic pregnancy, who requires admission and definitive treatment (Gilling-Smith et al. 1994).

D *Disadvantages* (**differential diagnosis**): a speculum examination may be performed in order to visualize the os, some women will decline this, viewing such examinations as increasing the risk of miscarriage, although there is no evidence to support this.

It is important that privacy is ensured for gynaecological examinations in a busy ED and that a chaperone is present throughout the procedure.

Although dealing with the physical symptoms is of great importance, the level of anxiety that a woman may experience should not be underestimated and the nurse must offer support and information. Other causes of PV bleeding are highlighted in Box 6.1.

Miscarriage: treatment and pathophysiology

In threatened miscarriage there is bleeding into the choriodecidual space. The cervical os will remain closed, however, careful monitoring of the patient is necessary as increased and profuse vaginal bleeding can occur at any time.

There are several outcomes of a threatened miscarriage: the bleeding settles spontaneously and the pregnancy proceeds uneventfully to full term with the delivery of a healthy infant. However, profuse bleeding can occur at any time and this may be accompanied by severe, painful, rhythmic uterine contractions. This is termed an inevitable miscarriage and, as the term implies, loss of the pregnancy is inevitable. In this situation there is dilatation of the cervix, on speculum examination, products of conception may be seen in the cervical os and should be removed with sponge forceps as they can cause pain and cervical dilatation which can result in a severe vasovagal reaction. The management is resuscitation using an ABC approach as the woman may present with profuse vaginal bleeding and be haemodynamically compromised as a result. Intravenous fluids must be commenced and in some cases a blood transfusion may be necessary. If bleeding is severe and continuous, Ergometrine 0.25–0.5 mg should be administered intravenously. An inevitable miscarriage can result in either a complete or incomplete miscarriage. A complete miscarriage is when all the products of conception have been expelled and the bleeding and pain subside along with a closed cervical os.

Ultrasound scan will reveal an empty uterus. A woman may be discharged from the ED following a complete miscarriage and it is therefore important that clinicians are aware of the practical advice and follow-up which should be given (Box 6.3).

Box 6.3   Information following miscarriage

- Bleeding may last up to two weeks but should gradually decrease
- Sanitary pads should be used to reduce the risk of infection; avoid tampons until next period.
- If bleeding becomes heavy and/or offensive, seek medical advice – this could indicate retained products of conception or infection.
- The next period should be within 4–6 weeks.
- Sexual intercourse should not be resumed until the bleeding settles to again reduce the risk of infection. Should sexual intercourse take place, a condom should be used.
- Although couples may feel anxious and depressed about the miscarriage, they will still need to be advised with regard to contraception – hormonal methods of contraception can be started immediately but the diaphragm will need to be checked 4 weeks after the miscarriage and should not be relied upon in the meantime.
- The Miscarriage Association can offer advice and time to talk and details of the Association should be given if the couple would like this information
- Rest is advised and she should stay off work for two weeks.
- Future pregnancies should be discussed sensitively – it is usually advised that couples wait until after the next period although a few months may be suggested.
- Rhesus negative women should be given Anti-D.

Incomplete miscarriage results in continued, profuse bleeding and again severe pain from uterine contractions. Not all products of conception have been expelled and it is usually the placenta that is retained. The management and care are the same as for an inevitable miscarriage and the woman will need to be prepared for surgery where an evacuation of retained products of conception (ERPC) will be performed.

Infection can be a sequela of miscarriage, this can often result from an incomplete miscarriage and the woman presents as febrile, with an increased pulse rate, tachypnoea and hypotension. Abdominal tenderness is present: the infection may be confined to the products of conception, alternatively, spread of infection can lead to endometritis, salpingitis, peritonitis and septicaemia. In this instance swabs and blood cultures should be taken. The woman will require rapid resuscitation, intravenous antibiotic administration, and careful monitoring of urinary output. Other complications include circulatory failure, and rarely a perforated or gangrenous uterus.

Ectopic pregnancy

> **Scenario 6.2** Ectopic pregnancy
>
> Juliet is a 24-year-old who is admitted to the ED with moderate pain in her lower abdomen, non-colicky in nature, along with right-sided abdominal tenderness for two weeks increasing in the last 24 hours. She has some brown vaginal loss and is amenorrhoeic with her last menstrual period being seven weeks ago. Her pulse is 90/minute and blood pressure is 110/70 mmHg.
>
> Juliet's condition has been stable since admission when she suddenly complains of a sudden increase in pain within her abdomen and of feeling faint. Recordings show that she is now hypotensive, with an increase in her pulse rate to 120 bpm. Her skin becomes clammy and she complains of dizziness. Juliet has severe abdominal pain; abdominal distension and shoulder tip pain.

D *Data* (scientific facts): from the primary data gathered, Juliet is presenting with abdominal pain and tenderness. According to Weckstein et al. (1995) in most situations, an ectopic pregnancy is not easy to diagnose clinically and a high index of suspicion should be maintained. A woman admitted with such symptoms needs a prompt diagnosis to be made in order to prevent complications occurring. Initially Juliet was not in a collapsed state and while she was experiencing moderate pain, she was haemodynamically stable. The patient may present with sudden onset of symptoms or a more gradual course (Pitkin et al. 2003). Juliet's condition should be closely monitored, as ectopic pregnancy remains a major cause of maternal death, partly due to the difficulty in diagnosis. Cox et al. (2003) emphasize that the diagnosis of ectopic pregnancy should be considered in all women of reproductive age with abdominal pain, vaginal bleeding or collapse. Assessment of airway, breathing and circulation (ABC) must be carefully undertaken with continuous monitoring of haemodynamic status and vaginal blood loss. The level of pain should be assessed and monitored and intravenous access should be established early.

Prior to any pelvic examination, if ectopic pregnancy is expected, it is wise to site an intravenous line as rupture of the ectopic may occur during the examination; gentle pelvic examination may reveal cervical excitation pain, because the tube is distorted by the enlarging ectopic pregnancy.

Serum beta human chorionic gonadotrophin (HCG) is of more value than urinary HCG as an ectopic pregnancy may not produce enough HCG to provide a positive result. An ultrasound scan may identify a tubal gestational sac. In a woman who presents in this way a laparoscopy will be performed in order to plan appropriate treatment.

Juliet's condition suddenly deteriorates and clearly tubal rupture has occurred. The two priorities in management are to resuscitate Juliet due to haemorrhagic shock, while at the same time prepare her for surgery. Immediate laparotomy is necessary to control haemorrhage (Pitkin et al. 2003). A senior registrar should be called. High flow oxygen by mask should be administered, bloods must be taken for haemoglobin estimation, full blood count, urea and electrolytes and six units of blood should be cross-matched. Collapse due to ruptured ectopic pregnancy can happen very suddenly with rapid deterioration in the woman's condition. Until surgery is performed the woman will continue to bleed profusely, hence rapid fluid replacement is essential. Abdominal pain is usually severe with abdominal distension occurring. The patient should be transferred urgently to theatre and time should not be wasted in trying to get a scan. Laparotomy will be performed in this instance along with salpingectomy, or salpingostomy; conservation of the tube may take place where possible.

In managing the woman with a ruptured ectopic pregnancy the key point is to resuscitate while making urgent arrangements for theatre (Cox et al. 2003).

E *Emotions* (intuition): early diagnosis of an ectopic pregnancy is vital in order to prevent further damage to the tube, reduce the likelihood of maternal death, and to preserve fertility. This is particularly important, as ectopic pregnancy can be difficult to diagnose, resembling other conditions such as appendicitis, rupture or torsion of an ovarian cyst and serious consequences can occur if it is missed. Remembering Lewis and Chamberlain's (1989) triad of pain, vaginal bleeding and amenorrhoea can assist in the diagnosis.

A *Advantages*: the following points are crucial to the diagnosis and management of a woman with an ectopic pregnancy:

- When a fertile woman presents with abdominal pain, always consider ectopic pregnancy.
- If any fertile woman faints, assume that she could be exsanguinating from a ruptured ectopic pregnancy.
- ßHCG should be performed, even if she has not missed a period.
- The woman may not present with typical symptoms.
- Positive ßHCG + empty uterus = ectopic pregnancy.

Women presenting to the ED of childbearing age with unexplained abdominal pain should have ectopic pregnancy excluded as part of their management. Urinalysis for HCG is now quick, easy and sensitive.

D *Disadvantages* (**differential diagnoses**): there can be difficulty in diagnosing this condition, Negating the primary diagnosis is essential as a delay or misdiagnosis can lead to maternal death. Haemorrhage in ruptured ectopic pregnancies can be severe due the large blood supply to the uterus.

Box 6.4 Ectopic pregnancy

Ectopic pregnancy affects one in every 80–100 pregnancies (RCOG 2002). It is a life-threatening condition and a gynaecological emergency. Ectopic, or extra-uterine pregnancy, is when the fertilized ovum implants outside the uterine cavity and in any tissue other than the endometrium. The commonest sites include the fallopian tube, the ovary, the cervix and rarely the abdominal cavity. Normally the ovum will be fertilized in the ampulla of the fallopian tube and will embed in the deciduas of the uterus after completing its developmental journey along the fallopian tube, ready for implantation in the uterine cavity. According to Lewis and Chamberlain (1989), if there is any delay in the passage of the fertilised ovum along the tube, the development of the trophoblast may be so advanced that it begins to embed.

The patient may complain of central or localized lower abdominal pain.. The period of amenorrhoea is commonly between six and eight weeks; there may be frank red vaginal bleeding and more commonly, brown vaginal loss. Vaginal bleeding occurs as the decidua sloughs after the demise of the foetus (Pitkin et al. 2003).

The pain from a growing ectopic pregnancy is due to localized distension of the tube; when tubal rupture occurs, there is intraperitoneal bleeding and the pain becomes continuous and more severe. The degree of shock depends on the amount of intraperitoneal haemorrhage. Shoulder tip pain occurs due to blood making contact with the diaphragm, subsequently cardiopulmonary collapse occurs. The term 'tubal rupture' refers to cases in which the wall of the tube gives way as a result of erosion by the trophoblast and increased tension in the tube (Lewis and Chamberlain 1989). In some cases ectopic pregnancy will spontaneously resolve, either by tubal abortion or tubal re-absorption.

The diagnosis of ectopic pregnancy can be very difficult in some instances. The Report on Confidential Enquiries into Maternal and Child Health (Lewis and Drife 2002) revealed that the rate of deaths from ectopic pregnancies has not declined since 1993. Clearly the need for accurate diagnosis and treatment is essential.

Obstetric haemorrhage

Bleeding in late pregnancy can be due to ante-partum haemorrhage (APH), defined as bleeding from the 24th week of pregnancy until the onset of labour. Intra-partum haemorrhage refers to bleeding from the onset of labour until the end of the second stage and post-partum haemorrhage to bleeding from the third stage of labour until the end of the puerperium. Ante-partum haemorrhage (APH) can be due to either placenta praevia or abruptio placentae. Other possible local causes are listed in Box 6.5.

Box 6.5   Local causes of APH

- Polyp
- Cervical ectopy
- Cervicitis
- Cervical carcinoma (although this can occur in pregnancy, it is quite rare)
- Vulval varicosities
- Trauma
- Infection
- 'Show' of labour
- Vasa praevia

Non-pregnant causes of vaginal bleeding

There are a number of causes of vaginal bleeding, which are not related to pregnancy, these include: uterine fibroids, trauma, infection and malignancy. While pregnancy must always be considered and excluded, women can experience profuse haemorrhage from these conditions.

Ovarian cysts

Scenario 6.3 Ovarian cyst
Rajwinder is a 36-year-old woman admitted with a history of sudden onset of unilateral lower abdominal pain which is sharp, colicky and intense in nature. She is nauseated and has vomited once since admission. She describes a slight vaginal blood loss. Her respiratory rate is 24, pulse rate is 102 bpm and blood pressure is 120/75 mm Hg. Rajwinder is apyrexial.

D *Data* (scientific facts): from the primary data gathered, Rajwinder's vital signs could indicate slight compensation or they could reflect the pain and anxiety she is feeling. The nature and intensity of her abdominal pain suggest an acute abdominal condition and emergency care should consist of assessment of airway, breathing and circulation, along with the provision of supplemental oxygen and oximetric monitoring. Intravenous access should be established. As Rajwinder has severe, colicky lower abdominal pain, associated with vomiting, torsion of an ovarian cyst must be considered. Pain may be intermittent as the cyst twists and untwists; a mass may enlarge acutely as the veins in its pedicle become obstructed.

   Pain assessment and monitoring are vital: analgesia should be titrated to pain and an anti-emetic administered. Recurrent nausea and vomiting can occur and is due to a vagal response to a twisted, stretched mesentery. This presentation can be similar to ectopic pregnancy, it is therefore, vital to determine pregnancy status by urinary or serum HCG testing. Vaginal spotting may occur secondary to decreased oestrogen levels and to hormonal imbalances.

E *Emotions* (intuition): the presenting symptoms indicate a surgical emergency and early recognition of the severity of Rajwinder's condition is important as symptoms can become life-threatening or further complications occur. Care and sensitivity are needed as the outcome can affect any future fertility.

A *Advantages*: if the woman is haemodynamically stable, an ultrasound scan can be performed to aid diagnosis. Bloods should be taken for haemoglobin estimation (anaemia may be present if there has been haemorrhaging from repeated twisting and untwisting of the pedicle), full blood count (the white cell count may be normal or elevated), urea and electrolytes and group and x-match, as intraperitoneal haemorrhage may also occur. Torsion of an ovarian cyst is a very serious condition and requires surgical intervention. Early preparation for surgery is essential to relieve pain and also aid the possibility of ovarian conservation; however, either oophorectomy or salpingo-oophorectomy may be performed. Early referral to a gynaecologist is essential to expedite the patient's definitive care.

D *Disadvantages* (**differential diagnosis**): other possible serious disorders which need to be excluded are ectopic pregnancy, appendicitis, pelvic inflammatory disease and diverticulitis.

Box 6.6 Ovarian cysts and complications

There are a number of gynaecological conditions that can affect the function of the ovaries which include:

- Cysts
- Cancer.

Ovarian cysts are fluid-filled sacs or pockets within or on the surface of an ovary. They can affect women of all ages and although they are initially benign, there is the potential for malignant change. Simple ovarian cysts are usually follicular or corpus luteum in origin. There are a number of other histological types of ovarian cysts. Ovarian cysts in the early stages of development are often asymptomatic but symptoms, if any, include dull pelvic pain, delayed menstruation followed by irregular or heavier than normal bleeding.

Ovarian cysts are common; however, complications do arise and can cause severe symptoms, which are potentially life-threatening (Cox et al. 2003).

According to Cox et al., emergency surgical management of an ovarian cyst is usually required because of a cyst accident as the patient presents with symptoms due to one of the following: torsion, haemorrhage, rupture or infection.

Rupture can cause excruciating pain levels and requires immediate surgery. The treatment usually involves ovarian cystectomy.

Torsion is the most common complication of ovarian tumours (Govan and Garrey 1985). Torsion can occur with any type of ovarian tumour and is particularly likely if the woman has a dermoid cyst (a benign germ cell tumour containing tissue such as skin, hair, teeth, cartilage, gastrointestinal, respiratory and nervous tissue), as these develop long pedicles. Torsion results from complete or partial twisting of the ovarian pedicle, which can lead to ovarian necrosis. The veins carrying blood away from the ovary become obstructed but the arteries continue to deliver blood. This happens because veins are thin-walled structures and blood flow is impeded more easily than that inside the much thicker-walled arteries. This results in haemorrhage into the tumour and peritoneum, which if not controlled, will result in gangrene.

In summary, torsion of an ovarian cyst results in:

- twisting of its vascular stalk
- disruption of the blood supply
- subsequent necrosis and pain
- necessary surgical intervention.

Box 6.7 Causes of ovarian pain

Remember – 'THIN RIM'

- **T** – Torsion
- **H** – Haemorrhage
- **I** – Infection
- **N** – Necrosis
- **R** – Rupture
- **I** – Infarction
- **M** – Malignant change

(Cox et al. 2003)

Pelvic inflammatory disease

Scenario 6.4 Pelvic inflammatory disease

Donna Adams aged 16, presents with severe abdominal pain, which has been progressive over the last three days. She has experienced some pain and irregularities of menstruation recently.

She complains of lower abdominal pain and tenderness, which is worse on movement and a purulent, offensive vaginal discharge.

She is febrile (39.2°C) and tachycardic on admission.

D *Data* (**scientific facts**): From the primary data gathered, Donna presents as being systematically unwell and needs careful assessment of her general condition. An ABC approach must be taken with monitoring of vital signs. The temperature is raised in response to infection. Careful observation of any deterioration should be reported, in which case a laparoscopy may be performed and which allows direct specimen collection for culture. Intravenous fluids and antibiotics should be commenced. If systematically unwell, antibiotic cover is required for chlamydia and neisseria gonorrhoea and anaerobes, such as those from bacterial vaginosis (Cox et al. 2003). Endocervical, high vaginal and urethral swabs should be taken. Blood cultures may also be taken. Donna's menstrual cycle may be upset if inflammation of the ovaries is present as menstrual irregularities are common. In addition, it is possible that retrograde menstruation may cause an increase in symptoms during menstruation. Pain assessment and management are important as the type and site of pain may indicate the location of the infection. She should be carefully monitored for signs of peritonitis. Bloods will be taken for a full blood count and erythrocyte sedimentation rate.

E *Emotions* (**intuition**): the severity of symptoms should necessitate early and prompt treatment of which the aims are:

- to alleviate the pain and systemic malaise associated with infection;
- to achieve microbiological cure;
- to prevent development of permanent tubal damage with associated sequelae, such as chronic pelvic pain, ectopic pregnancy and infertility. Inadequately treated disease may progress to tubo-ovarian abscess (Rosevear 2002);
- to prevent the spread of infection to others. Follow-up should include a genito-urinary medicine referral.

If an intrauterine contraceptive device is in situ, this should be removed.

A *Advantages*: even in the worst cases of PID the prognosis can be good if the diagnosis is made early and the patient is treated with appropriate antibiotics (Lewis and Chamberlain 1989).

D *Disadvantages* (**differential diagnoses**): accurate diagnosis can be difficult and a menstrual and contraceptive history is important, as the main differential diagnoses are ectopic pregnancy, ovarian cyst or accident, appendicitis, endometriosis, cystitis and complications of the intrauterine contraceptive device. If treatment is delayed and suppuration occurs in the tubes, the progress of the disease can usually be stopped and the formation of a pyosalpinx or pelvic abscess avoided, but the hope of restoration of fertility is poor (Lewis and Chamberlain 1989).

Box 6.8 Pelvic inflammatory disease (PID)

PID is an 'umbrella' term which encompasses any inflammatory condition of the female reproductive system, to include the cervix – cervicitis, endometrium – endometritis, parametrium – parametritis, fallopian tubes – salpingitis, ovaries – oophoritis, tubo-ovarian and pelvic abscess and peritonitis. Due to adhesions the bowel may be involved. Any organ or combination of organs may be affected, caused by bacterial infections (Lewis and Chamberlain 1989).

Upper genital tract infection or PID is a common gynaecological emergency which poses a major risk to female reproductive health.

Symptoms include:

- fever, foul-smelling vaginal discharge, lower abdominal pain, pain with coitus;

- If an abscess has developed, then a fluid-filled mass may be palpated.

Usually PID is caused by sexually transmitted micro-organisms that migrate from the vagina to the uterus, fallopian tubes and the ovaries. However, it may be as a result of ascending infection from gynaecological procedures such as termination of pregnancy. The intrauterine contraceptive device may also be associated with ascending infection.

Infection of the right tube and ovary can occur in appendicitis, or both tubes may be involved in pelvic peritonitis or abscess. The fallopian tubes in particular may become red and swollen and filled with pus.

Tubo-ovarian inflammatory masses can be a complication of PID which may require surgical drainage or salpingo-oophorectomy.

Box 6.9   Consequences of untreated pelvic inflammatory disease

- Chronic pelvic pain
- Abscess
- Peritonitis
- Adhesion formation
- Ectopic pregnancy
- Infertility – fibrosis associated with PID may cause tubal blockage

---

Emergency delivery

Scenario 6.5   Emergency delivery

You are called to the car park to assess Nicola, a 26-year-old who is 39/40 pregnant and has been having intense and regular uterine contractions. On arrival, Nicola is in the back seat of the car and is extremely anxious, you manage to persuade her to get onto a wheel chair and take her into the ED.

Nicola is accompanied by her husband and has not had any previous pregnancies.

D *Data* (scientific facts): it is difficult for a nulliparous woman to understand the sensations (including sometimes severe pain) that she will experience during childbirth until they actually occur (Steer and Flint 1999). Nicola is presenting in established labour and assessment of the frequency and intensity of the uterine contractions suggests that delivery appears imminent. It is likely that Nicola will complain of a 'bearing down feeling' or urgency to defecate. If the baby is not crowning, or if the mother is not yet completely dilated, and no complications are noted, the mother may be moved to the obstetric ward (Benzoni 2006).

Preparations should be made and a delivery pack opened, a midwife and/or obstetrician should be called. A rapid, but thorough, ABC assessment should be made and maternal vital signs should be recorded every 10 minutes. Shock should be treated as necessary and intravenous access established if indicated.

A rapid obstetric history should be obtained which includes: the woman's age; reproductive history to include last normal menstrual period; parity and estimated date of expected delivery; obstetric care received during the pregnancy; the number of previous pregnancies and previous births (to include complications); any medical problems (to include hypertension and oedema); and, last, any medications or allergies. The onset of contractions and pain including frequency, intensity and duration should be determined, along with the amount and colour of vaginal bleeding and discharge and evidence of rupture of the amniotic sac.

Physical examination will include inspection, auscultation and palpation of the abdomen to assess the uterine size, tone and contractility, duration of contractions and the time between contractions, the foetal lie and position, and foetal heart. According to Benzoni (2006), if the baby is not crowning (i.e. child's head bulging at the perineum), a brief vaginal examination, performed with a sterile-gloved hand, will reveal if the cervix is dilated (to 10cm) and/or effaced (thinned to about 1mm). The practitioner should assist with the delivery process and should position the woman comfortably.

Drapes should be applied and principles of asepsis adhered to. Box 6.10 outlines the procedure for emergency delivery.

E *Emotions* (**intuition**): the emergency practitioner should remain calm and offer a reassuring and supportive approach to the woman and her partner, who are likely to be very anxious. Patients will usually have a detailed birthing plan and may be distressed about not being able to follow it as they will have been preparing mentally for this moment for some time.

Support for both the patient and her partner is essential, an emergency delivery can be a traumatic and emotional experience for all involved.

A *Advantages*: recommendations for emergency departments are that all pregnant women that present should be seen quickly, by a doctor, and those with anything other than very minor physical injuries should be seen in conjunction with an obstetrician or senior midwife (Lewis and Drife 2002). If these are not available on site, then arrangements should be made with the local maternity unit to discuss these cases.

D *Disadvantages* (**differential diagnoses**): the priority in this scenario is to make a rapid ABCDE assessment of the mother while summoning expert

Box 6.10   Emergency delivery

- When the infant's head appears during crowning, place fingers on bony part of skull. Exert very gentle pressure to prevent rapid delivery and allow infant's head to emerge slowly.
- Once the head is delivered, a finger should be gently passed to detect if the umbilical cord is wrapped around the baby's neck. If the cord is felt, it should be slipped over the baby's head; if the cord is tight and it cannot be slipped over the infant's head, place umbilical clamps 2 inches apart and cut the cord between the clamps. If this happens, it is important to proceed with the delivery as quickly as possible.
- When the head is delivered, wipe the infant's face and suction nose and mouth to minimize any aspiration of amniotic fluid and blood. *It is extremely important to check for meconium in the amniotic fluid during and post delivery*. Aspiration can create life-threatening respiratory complications.
- While supporting infant's head, deliver the shoulders with the next contraction. The posterior shoulder follows the anterior shoulder and the remainder of the baby's body should follow.
- Clamp umbilical cord between two clamps and cut the cord between them as pulsations cease.
- Dry and wrap infant to minimize heat loss.
- Assess the infant's APGAR score.
- Let placenta deliver normally. Note: do not pull on cord.
- Keep the placenta covered in a receptacle.
- Place sterile pad over vulva, assess and monitor vital signs and vaginal loss post-delivery. Treat for shock if necessary.
- Place the mother in a comfortable position after delivery and allow contact between the two.
- Record time of delivery.
- Transport to delivery unit.

assistance to enable an assessment of the unborn baby. If labour has been prolonged, foetal distress may be present. In this case emergency delivery by caesarean section may be indicated. Following vaginal delivery, post-partum haemorrhage must be negated, regular observations should be carried out and the perineum should be observed for signs of trauma. The baby should be given an ABC assessment by a trained member of staff and treated appropriately.

Box 6.11 Labour and delivery

Labour is the process by which the foetus is expelled from the uterus and is defined as the onset of regular, painful contractions with progressive cervical effacement and dilatation of the cervix accompanied by descent of the presenting part.

Labour can be divided into three stages. The first stage of labour can be defined as the time from onset of labour to full dilatation of the cervix (10cm). The second stage describes the time from full dilatation of the cervix to delivery of the foetus. The third stage is the time from delivery of the foetus until delivery of the placenta (Baker 2006).

Pitkin et al. (2003) describe the signs of placental separation as comprising:

- lengthening of the umbilical cord
- a gush of blood vaginally
- firming of the fundus.

Conclusion

This chapter has discussed some of the gynaecological and obstetric emergencies that practitioners may encounter. Unfortunately the full range of such emergencies has not been discussed within the scope of this chapter but it is hoped that the information presented will enable practitioners to manage women effectively, resulting in more positive outcomes where possible.

7 Acute surgical emergencies

Paul Newcombe

Introduction

The focus of this chapter is acute surgical emergencies affecting the abdominal/gastrointestinal (GI) system – the 'acute abdomen'. Figure 7.1 shows essential anatomy and physiology (A&P), but readers are referred to A&P texts to supplement this (Marieb and Hoehn 2007). Common acute surgical presentations are explored with reference to pathophysiology, and how this manifests in clinical and vital signs. Emphasis is on rapid, but thorough patient assessment, history taking and data collection. Timely initial resuscitation, early symptom relief and acute management are the interventional focus, but references are also made to definitive management options such as surgery.

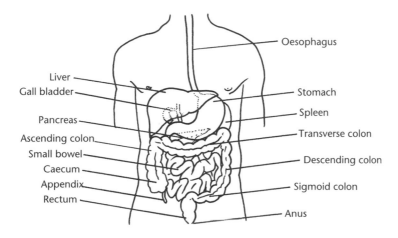

Figure 7.1 The gastrointestinal system

Patient assessment

An accurate history is vital for reaching a differential diagnosis in acute surgical emergencies. The commonest presenting complaint is abdominal pain, however, there may be other predominant symptoms such as vomiting, diarrhoea, constipation or collapse. Abdominal pathology should also be considered in presentations of chest pain, back pain, shoulder pain and genitalia pain.

Abdominal pain

If abdominal pain is present, and a useful method of exploring this is the PQRST mnemonic (Albarran 2002) (Box 7.1), although it was originally designed for assessment of chest pain, this tool is easily transferable.

Box 7.1 PQRST mnemonic
P – Precipitating factors **Q** – Quality **R** – Region and radiation **S** – Severity and associated symptoms **T** – Timing and treatment

Precipitating factors
Suitable questions include, 'What were you doing when the pain started?' and, 'Can you identify anything which has caused this pain or made it worse?' The patient may have experienced the pain after eating, for example.

Quality
What does the pain feel like? Encourage patients to describe the nature of the pain in their own words. Possible descriptions include cramping, sharp, burning, aching, boring and throbbing. The significance of this character is very important (Table 7.1).

Region and radiation
Encourage the patient to indicate the location(s) of pain as specifically as possible, however, the pain may be poorly localized. Also enquire if pain radiates elsewhere, such as chest, back, shoulder or genitals (Table 7.1). The location of the pain may have moved and this is likely to be significant. Use the quadrant or segmental system when documenting the location(s) of pain (Figure 7.2).

Severity and associated symptoms
The level of pain should be assessed using a validated pain assessment tool. There are many associated symptoms, which require specific exploration, such

Table 7.1 Types of abdominal pain

Visceral pain	Parietal (somatic) pain	Referred (radiating) pain
• Stretching, inflammation, ischaemia or contraction of a hollow viscus or organ, such as bowel, gall bladder, ureters and uterus • Described as a dull ache, cramping or colic. Comes in waves • Difficult to localize. Generally in the midline and epigastric, periumbilical or suprapubic area. May radiate to a specific site • Often accompanied by non-specific symptoms, such as nausea, anorexia and diaphoresis • Not aggravated by movement	• Parietal peritoneum is better innervated by pain fibres • Pain described as sharp, stabbing or burning • Easily localized due to irritation or inflammation of parietal peritoneum • Aggravated by movement and palpation	• Pain is felt at a distance from the source • Diseased or injured organ shares nerve pathway with another area • Common examples include shoulder tip pain due to phrenic nerve stimulation, caused by irritation of the diaphragm with blood or air following rupture of an abdominal organ; loin to groin pain in renal colic

Source: Adopted from Epstein et al. (2003)

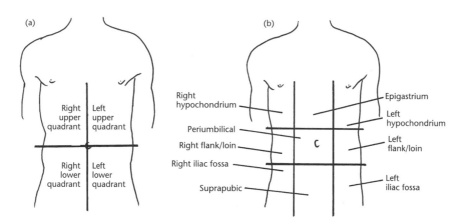

Figure 7.2 Anatomical areas of the abdomen: (a) quadrants; (b) segments

as nausea, vomiting, diarrhoea and fever. Clues from the history thus far will prompt the practitioner on what to enquire about further. These associated symptoms are discussed below.

Timing and treatment

The time-course can be gained by exploring when the symptoms started, if the onset was sudden or gradual, how long it lasted and if it is constant or intermittent. Has the patient taken anything for their symptoms, such as over-the-counter medications? Did it provide any relief? It is also important to enquire if there is anything else that makes the pain better, such as eating, opening the bowels or changing position.

Nausea and vomiting

Nausea is a common non-specific symptom of illness and is particularly common with gastrointestinal illness. If there is a history or evidence of vomiting, then investigation into the amount, frequency and nature of the vomitus is essential. Of particular importance is presence of blood in the vomit. This may be fresh, bright red blood indicating recent upper gastrointestinal bleeding, or old blood described as 'coffee grounds'. The patient may also describe vomiting altered food or bile. In advanced large bowel obstruction the patient may vomit faecal liquid.

Anorexia

This is another non-specific indicator of illness, but again loss of appetite is common with gastrointestinal disorders, and is particularly likely if nausea and/or vomiting are present.

Weight loss

Both the amount of weight lost and over what time frame should be estimated. Whether this was intentional or not should also be ascertained. Significant unintentional weight loss is a sinister sign suggesting malignancy.

Indigestion

It is important to explore what the patient means by this, as there are various descriptions for these common symptoms such as reflux, heartburn and dyspepsia. It is not uncommon for cardiac pain to be described as indigestion.

Dysphagia

Difficulty swallowing may be caused by three main factors: a problem with the complex neural control of swallowing, oesophageal stricture or direct obstruction due to a tumour, for example. Odynophagia refers to pain or discomfort on swallowing.

Bowel symptoms

Normal bowel habits range from more than once a day to less than once a week. If there is a history of constipation, then the time of 'bowels last open' (BLO) should be recorded. If there is a history of diarrhoea, then the frequency should be estimated, and the nature described – loose, watery or containing mucus. Specific enquiries should be made about the presence of blood in the stool. If the response is positive, then again the volume should be estimated, and the nature described. Fresh blood indicates lower GI bleeding, such as haemorrhoids. Malaena is a characteristic black, sticky, offensive smelling liquid, which indicates upper GI bleeding.

Wind

Despite constipation the patient should still report passing flatus. If they are not, this indicates bowel obstruction. Excessive belching may indicate obstruction, and hiccups may indicate perforation as a result of diaphragmatic irritation.

Distension

The patient may describe this as feeling bloated. However, distension might only be detected upon physical examination. The causes for abdominal distension can be remembered as the five Fs (Box 7.2).

Box 7.2 Causes of distension: the five Fs
• Fat
• Fluid
• Faeces
• Flatus
• Foetus

Genitourinary symptoms

A common cause of lower abdominal pain in women is urinary tract infection (UTI). Enquire about burning pain on passing urine (dysuria), frequency or urgency, passing small volumes of urine and offensive smelling urine. Women should also be asked about gynaecological symptoms, such as vaginal bleeding or discharge. Men should be asked about testicular pain and urethral discharge. UTI is not common in men. A recent sexual history should be gained from both sexes.

Fever

Mild fever is an indication of an inflammatory response and is commonly seen in acute surgical emergencies. A higher fever indicates an infective process, and when associated with signs of shock, suggests sepsis (Chapter 2). Fever is common in conditions such as appendicitis, cholecystitis and peritonitis

General malaise

This is another non-specific indicator of illness and includes signs such as lethargy, listlessness and feeling generally unwell.

Respiratory/cardiovascular symptoms

The patient should also be asked about shortness of breath, dizziness and chest pain, particularly if abdominal aortic aneurysm (AAA) is suspected.

Past medical history

A history of ischaemic heart disease will require the practitioner to exclude this as a cause of current symptoms through appropriate investigations, such as ECG and cardiac enzymes (Chapter 3). Further cardiovascular history, such as hypertension, should raise the suspicion of AAA. Surgical history is important to document, particularly if the patient has had any previous operations. Other relevant history includes previous problems with any of the abdominal system, for example, liver, kidneys, bowel, pancreas and any other significant co-morbidity, such as clotting disorders, anaemia, and cancer. The female patient should be asked about previous obstetric and gynaecological history.

Drug history

There are many drugs, which affect the abdominal system, either directly or via side effects. Antibiotics commonly cause diarrhoea, and some are nephrotoxic, such as vancomycin. Opiates can cause nausea and constipation. Non-steroidal anti-inflammatory drugs such as diclofenac, ibuprofen and aspirin can damage the gut mucosa and cause gastrointestinal bleeding. They are also nephrotoxic when taken over long periods, or with existing renal impairment. Patients with a history of GI bleeding should be specifically asked about anti-coagulant medications, such as warfarin. Iron supplements produce black stool not dissimilar to malaena. Enquiring about allergies to medicine is always important if the patient is to be prescribed anything, but also some allergic reactions can include GI symptoms, such as nausea, vomiting and abdominal pain.

Social and family history

The patient's age will greatly influence the potential diagnosis, and also their response to illness. Recent foreign travel should be noted, particularly to areas where diseases such as malaria, hepatitis and GI disorders are common. History of appropriate immunizations and prophylactic medication (or not) should also be recorded. Alcohol is a known toxin to the GI system and consumption should be estimated. Excess intake can damage the gut mucosa and cause GI bleeding. Alcohol is also one of the two commonest causes of pancreatitis. However, alcohol's most devastating effects are exerted upon the liver. Cirrhosis causes oesophageal varices, clotting disorders, jaundice, ascites, encephalopathy and ultimately liver failure. History of illicit drug use should also be sought; for example, heroin, as an opiate, produces side effects discussed previously. There are also inherent risks to the GI system with injecting drugs, such as transmission of hepatitis. Finally, significant family history should also be noted, particularly when there is a possible genetic link, such as cancer and inflammatory bowel disease.

Vital signs

General appearance
Does the patient look unwell? Are they alert? Are they distressed or in obvious discomfort? Do they look pale or dehydrated? Are they writhing or lying very still?

Respiratory
Measure the respiratory rate. Tachypnoea is an early indicator of shock, but may also be raised due to pain and anxiety. Respiratory effort may be restricted due to peritonitis, or diaphragmatic splinting caused by abdominal distension. Pulse oximetry should be used with caution in the shocked patient (Chapter 2).

Cardiovascular
Take a manual pulse. A weak, thready pulse is an indicator of shock. This is likely to be hypovolaemic shock in the surgical patient, but a fast, bounding pulse is an early sign of septic shock. Tachycardia is also a sign of pain and anxiety. Capillary refill time should be measured, noting skin temperature and evidence of diaphoresis. Record the blood pressure, and assess for indicators of shock (Chapter 2). Measure bilateral blood pressure if AAA is suspected. Measure postural blood pressure if there is evidence of volume loss or dehydration.

Temperature

Measure the core temperature. As stated previously, there are many infective causes of surgical emergencies.

Abdominal examination

Inspection
Look at the general shape, contours and symmetry of the abdomen. The abdomen is normally slightly concave, but the proportion of body fat will influence this. The abdomen should move gently with respiration, but obvious peristaltic movements are not normal. In thin patients it may be possible to observe pulsation of the abdominal aorta in the epigastrium. Note the presence of distension, scars from previous operations, dilated veins, bruising, hernias or other unidentified lumps. Striae (stretch marks) may be present and indicate weight gain and subsequent loss, such as in pregnancy.

Auscultation
Each quadrant of the abdomen should be auscultated for normal bowel sounds (Figure 7.2). They may be high-pitched in the initial stages of bowel obstruction. Absent bowel sounds indicate the gut is not functioning properly. Auscultation can also be used to listen for bruit – the turbulent flow of blood through narrowed arteries in various parts of the abdomen.

Palpation
Ask the patient to identify where the pain is and begin light palpation away from this area to gain their trust. Observe the patient's face for discomfort, such as grimacing. Palpate each quadrant systematically, noting areas of tenderness. Deep palpation is used to explore areas of tenderness further and assess masses and organomegaly. Guarding is an involuntary protective contraction of the abdominal muscles surrounding inflamed peritoneum. Rebound tenderness also indicates inflammation of the peritoneum; this is when the examiner palpates an area of tenderness and then quickly removes their hand. If the patient experiences increased pain when the hand is removed this is described as rebound tenderness. Board-like rigidity is a cardinal sign of peritonitis and the onset of septic shock, inhibiting further examination.

Percussion
Percussing over the normal abdomen should produce a resonant note indicating the presence of air in the gut. A dull note indicates fluid or solid mass, such as over a full bladder or impacted colon. Percussion is used to assess organomegaly and detect ascites as the cause of distension. Percussion can also illicit rebound tenderness.

Rectal examination
An abdominal examination is considered incomplete without a digital rectal examination (DRE). Indeed, tenderness may only be elicited upon DRE. The anus is inspected for haemorrhoids, skin tags, fissures and fistulae. Next a lubricated, gloved finger is inserted into the rectum following the curve of the sacrum. The wall of the rectum is examined by rotating the finger, palpating the prostate/cervix anteriorly. On removal the gloved finger is inspected for faeces and/or blood.

Further investigations

There are many further investigations, which may be appropriate. Practitioners should be guided by information gained so far during the assessment:

- An early electrocardiograph (ECG) should be considered for many patients presenting with abdominal pain, but particularly any patient with epigastric pain or upper abdominal pain of unclear aetiology; patients with a history of ischaemic heart disease (IHD); and all elderly patients.
- Measure blood sugar level in all patients with abdominal symptoms. This is vital for patients with a history of diabetes. Diabetic ketoacidosis may present with abdominal pain and vomiting.
- Perform urinalysis and send for culture if appropriate. A pregnancy test should be performed on all women of childbearing age presenting with abdominal symptoms.
- Blood tests include full blood count (FBC), urea and electrolytes (U&E) and glucose. If there is evidence of an inflammatory process, a c-reactive protein (CRP) is indicated. Evidence of infection and fever indicates the need for blood cultures. Patients with a history or evidence of liver impairment need liver function tests (LFT) and clotting studies. Patients with a history of clotting disorders or taking anti-coagulants also require clotting studies. Patients with upper abdominal pain require a serum amylase level. As stated previously, cardiac enzymes may be appropriate for many patients. If surgery is likely, a group and save (G&S) or cross-match should be taken.
- Appropriate standard radiographical investigations include plain supine abdominal X-ray and erect chest X-ray. More specific investigations include computed tomography (CT), ultrasound scanning (USS) and intravenous urogram (IVU).

General initial management

Appropriate initial management will be dictated by the patient's clinical condition. Management for specific conditions will be discussed later.

- All patients in respiratory distress or with evidence of shock should be given high concentration oxygen via an oxygen mask and reservoir.
- Gain early intravenous (IV) access and draw blood for investigations. Administer IV fluids as history and/or clinical signs indicate.
- There is much debate about whether analgesia should be withheld until after a diagnosis has been made. The theory is that analgesia will mask symptoms and make diagnosis difficult. However, there is no evidence to support this practice, and the consensus is that withholding analgesia is therefore unethical (McHale and LoVecchio 2001; Pasero 2003). Have a low threshold for IV opiates; titrate to pain, respiratory rate and sedation.
- The patient should be advised not to eat or drink (NBM) until thorough medical assessment is complete, although sips of clear fluids may be permissible. Give anti-emetics for nausea or vomiting.

Appendicitis

> **Scenario 7.1** Appendicitis
>
> A 25-year-old woman attends the emergency department with severe right iliac fossa pain. The pain began the night before in the middle of her stomach and she feels nauseous. She reports two episodes of loose bowel motions.
> Her respiratory rate is 24, pulse 110bpm and she has a low-grade fever.

D *Data* (scientific facts): the nurse will need to take a thorough history detailing the course of symptoms and character of the pain. Past medical history will also need to be considered for previous similar episodes. Vital signs demonstrate an inflammatory response. The nurse should look for evidence of established shock. The history suggests appendicitis, but gynaecological causes will also need to be considered. Further data collection should include routine blood tests, urinalysis and physical examination.

E *Emotions* (intuition): the nurse is using pattern recognition from previous experience of patients with right iliac fossa pain. Applying critical thinking should alert the nurse that there are many differential diagnoses for this presenting complaint.

A *Advantages*: the nurse's initial role is in early symptom relief with analgesia and anti-emetics. Gaining IV access and blood tests will expedite care. Communication of findings with medical colleagues, or preferably the surgical team will facilitate a definitive management plan. The patient should be advised to remain NBM in the interim.

D *Disadvantages* (**differential diagnoses**): an early pregnancy test is vital to exclude ectopic pregnancy for this patient. Abdominal examination is the key to reaching a diagnosis in presentations of right iliac fossa pain.

Prevalence

Appendicitis is one of the commonest causes of an acute abdomen, and appendicectomy is one of the most commonly performed intra-abdominal surgical procedures. However, diagnosis can be challenging and it is estimated that in as many as 20 per cent of appendicectomies, a normal appendix is removed (Liang 2005). This is often considered acceptable when weighed against the considerable risks of missing a ruptured appendix. Appendicitis is commonest in children and young adults.

Aetiology and pathophysiology

The vermiform appendix is an 8cm blind tube attached to the caecum where the small and large bowel joins. The appendix has no known function, but can readily become inflamed. The cause of appendicitis is not always known, but blockage with a faecolith – small, hard faeces – is often implicated. Organisms invade the mucosa causing inflammation. Swelling rapidly increases pressure in a small space and blood supply to the mucosa is compromised. Subsequent necrosis to the tip and wall of the appendix leads to rupture. Perforation and leakage of bowel contents may be contained and result in local abscess formation, or may be diffuse and cause generalized peritonitis (Tjandra 2006).

Clinical features

Pain
Abdominal pain is one of the commonest symptoms of appendicitis, and a typical presentation tends to follow a predictable pattern. Visceral pain from early inflammation of the appendix is diffuse and central. Over the next few hours as the overlying peritoneum becomes irritated, pain migrates to the right iliac fossa (McBurney's point), becoming localized and more severe. Many patients do not demonstrate this classic presentation.

Anorexia
There may be a period prior to the onset of abdominal pain where the patient feels generally unwell and doesn't want to eat.

Nausea and vomiting

Nausea may be present early on and may progress to vomiting as inflammation worsens. Severe vomiting suggests another cause of symptoms such as gastroenteritis.

Diarrhoea

It is not uncommon for patients with appendicitis to report loose stools. This is probably due to the inflamed appendix irritating the bowel mucosa. Severe diarrhoea may suggest alternative diagnoses, such as gastroenteritis or inflammatory bowel disease.

Fever

As appendicitis is an inflammatory condition, patients often complain of feeling mildly feverish. Significant fever may indicate perforation and peritonitis, or a different diagnosis.

Assessment

Vital signs

Subtle signs of an inflammatory response may be picked up from the patient's initial observations such as raised respiratory rate, mild tachycardia and low-grade fever. Significant tachycardia and hypotension suggest established shock as a result of perforation and peritonitis. Body temperature has been shown to be a poor indicator of appendicitis in some studies (Cardall et al. 2004).

Abdominal examination

Tenderness on palpation at McBurney's point is the key feature of appendicitis. The patient may also demonstrate guarding and rebound tenderness, and there may be right-sided tenderness on DRE. There are a number of additional specific tests, which can be employed to illicit tenderness from an inflamed appendix:

- Pain in the right lower quadrant when the left lower quadrant is palpated (Rovsing's sign).
- Pain exacerbated by resisted flexion of the right hip (psoas sign).
- Pain exacerbated by passive internal rotation of the right hip (obturator sign).

Generalized tenderness and rigidity suggest perforation and peritonitis. In delayed presentation, a ruptured appendix with subsequent abscess formation may produce a tender, palpable mass in the right iliac fossa (Tjandra

2006). Vaginal examination may be indicated to help exclude a gynaecological cause of symptoms.

Laboratory investigations

Raised inflammatory markers, such as white blood count (WBC) and CRP are associated with appendicitis. The value of such tests in confirming the diagnosis of appendicitis has been questioned by some studies (Cardall et al. 2004). However, a small study by Birchley (2006) concluded that WBC and CRP are more effective in supporting a diagnosis of appendicitis when they are raised than excluding it when they are not.

Urinalysis

This may help exclude urinary tract infection, renal colic or ectopic pregnancy as differential diagnoses.

Radiography

Radiography is most useful in patients where the diagnosis of appendicitis is uncertain following history and examination. Plain supine abdominal X-ray is of little value in appendicitis, but may help exclude other differential diagnoses, such as bowel obstruction. This will be indicated if perforation is suspected as will an erect chest X-ray. Identification of appendicitis may be possible on ultrasound and it may assist in ruling out gynaecological causes of symptoms. Computed tomography (CT) is expensive and not always available, but also has a role in the diagnosis of appendicitis, including identifying other pathology. Lin et al. (2005) found that CT scan is effective in identifying appendiceal rupture and masses. CT can also facilitate percutaneous drainage of an abscess.

Management

Early analgesics and anti-emetics may be required, and IV access should be gained. Once a diagnosis is reached, the patient will need to be prepared for theatre. They should be NBM and have IV fluids. Open appendicectomy via a characteristic incision is the usual operative management. This may be performed laparoscopically. Where the diagnosis is still unclear, the patient may be observed for 12–24 hours.

Cholecystitis

Acute cholecystitis is another of the most common surgical emergencies. Indeed, the gall bladder is the second most common organ requiring surgical intervention after the appendix. Medical folklore suggests that the risk of having gallstones can be identified by the five Fs: fair, fat, female, febrile and fifties. Certainly the incidence of gallstones is much higher in women and it increases with age.

Anatomy and physiology

The gall bladder is a pear-shaped sac, which lies on the inferior surface of the liver. Its neck opens into the cystic duct, which combines with the common hepatic duct to form the common bile duct. Before it reaches the sphincter of Oddi, where it joins the duodenum, it is joined by the pancreatic duct. The role of the gall bladder is to store excess bile produced by the liver and concentrate it by removing excess water and salt. Ingestion of fatty food stimulates the gall bladder to contract and secrete bile. Bile is a yellow/green solution containing a variety of substances such as bile salts and bile pigments. Bile salts emulsify fats. The main bile pigment is bilirubin. This is a waste product of haemoglobin recycling performed by the liver. Metabolism of bilirubin to urobilinogen gives faeces its brown colour. Excess bilirubin in the blood causes jaundice. This may occur in blockage to the outflow of bile or in liver disease (Marieb and Hoehn 2007).

Aetiology and pathophysiology

Gallstones are very common, with the majority being made up of cholesterol. In acute cholecystitis, blockage to the outflow of bile with a gallstone initiates an inflammatory process. Water continues to be absorbed from the bile contained within the gall bladder. This concentrated bile causes a chemical inflammation. The bile then usually becomes infected and this fuels the inflammatory process. The gall bladder swells and becomes oedematous. Further progression leads to a collection of pus, called empyema, and inflammation of surrounding structures. The blood supply to the gall bladder can become compromised, leading to necrosis and subsequent rupture. Perforation can cause peritonitis, local abscess or fistula formation.

Gallstones can also cause a blockage to the outflow of bile in the absence of infection. This is called biliary colic and symptoms can be similar to those of cholecystitis. Pain tends to be less severe, fever is absent and symptoms should resolve spontaneously after a short while. Recurrence of biliary colic is common, and the patient may go on to develop cholecystitis. Chronic cholecystitis occurs due to repeated attacks of obstruction and results in chronic inflammation of the gall bladder. Obstruction of the biliary tree and other causes may also result in infected bile – called acute cholangitis. This can prove fatal due to sepsis, kidney and liver failure (Habib and Canelo 2005).

Clinical features

Pain
Abdominal pain is a key feature of acute cholecystitis. Dull pain may begin in the epigastrium and swiftly localize to the right upper quadrant. Pain then tends to be severe, described as sharp and exacerbated by movement or deep breathing. Eating, which stimulates contraction of the gall bladder, may also exacerbate pain.

Nausea and vomiting
GI symptoms are common in cholecystitis. Nausea and anorexia are usually present, frequently accompanied by vomiting.

Fever
As an inflammatory process, fever is likely to be present. This may worsen as the condition progresses.

Jaundice
In severe cases, blockage to the outflow of bile causes bilirubin to build up in the blood and leak into the interstitial spaces. Mild jaundice is often best seen in the white of the eye (sclera).

Assessment

Vital signs
Similarly to appendicitis, the observations are likely to demonstrate an inflammatory response. Tachypnoea, tachycardia and a fever may all be present. Respiratory effort may be compromised by pain.

Abdominal examination
The patient is very likely to be tender in the right upper quadrant, with guarding and rebound tenderness. The gall bladder is not usually palpable. A specific test for cholecystitis is Murphy's sign. The patient takes a deep breath while the examiner palpates the right upper quadrant. The inflamed gall bladder moves down with inspiration and on contact with the examiner's hand the patient experiences acute tenderness and stops inspiration. In empyema or abscess formation a mass may be palpable under the right costal margin.

Laboratory investigations
Inflammatory markers are usually raised. Liver function tests (LFT) may be raised, particularly the bilirubin level. Amylase may also be slightly elevated.

Radiography

Ultrasound scan is the investigation of choice in cholecystitis. Gallstones may be identified, but a thickening of the gall bladder wall and surrounding fluid can make a diagnosis. Gallstones may also show up on abdominal X-ray. More invasive investigations include endoscopic retrograde cholangio-pancreatography (ERCP).

Management

Aim for early symptom relief with analgesics and anti-emetics. The patient should be NBM to rest the gut and prevent exacerbation of pain. Broad-spectrum IV antibiotics should be commenced as well as IV fluids if not drinking or volume depleted. Cholecystectomy was traditionally delayed while the condition was managed conservatively. However, a meta-analysis by Shikata et al. (2005) found that there was no benefit in delaying chole-cystectomy. Fagan et al. (2003) found this was particularly true for high-risk patients such as diabetics or those with a very high white cell count. Cholecystectomy is frequently performed laparoscopically.

Bowel obstruction

Bowel obstruction is another common surgical emergency and is divided into small and large bowel obstruction. Both either feature a blockage to the lumen or a failure of intestinal motility.

Anatomy and physiology

The small bowel is a 6m long narrow tube and comprises the duodenum, jejunum and ileum. It is a key site for digestion, aided by pancreatic enzymes and bile secreted into the duodenum. Faeces are liquid, as water absorption does not occur until the large bowel is reached. Most nutrient absorption occurs at the distal end of the ileum. The large bowel begins at the ileocaecal valve and includes the caecum, ascending colon, transverse colon, descending colon, sigmoid colon and rectum. It is just over a metre long and much wider than the small bowel. Ninety-five per cent of the water and sodium passing through the large intestine is reabsorbed and solid faeces are formed, aided by bacteria. Peristaltic contractions move faeces through the bowel. The blood supply to the bowel is via the mesenteric arteries. The nutrient rich blood is drained via the hepatic portal vein, where the liver removes nutrients for metabolism (Marieb and Hoehn 2007).

Aetiology and pathophysiology

Causes of obstruction vary depending on the level in the bowel. The commonest causes of small bowel obstruction are adhesions from previous surgery, strangulated hernias, malignancy, and volvulus – twisting of the bowel. Paralytic ileus may also occur in the small bowel, where the cause is lack of motility rather than mechanical obstruction. Large bowel obstruction is more common in the elderly and often caused by malignancy, but also by volvulus and diverticular disease. Constipation is often a feature, but rarely causes obstruction alone. Pseudo-obstruction is an ileus of the large bowel and also more common in the elderly. It is usually caused by an existing medical condition rather than mechanical obstruction, but clinical features are similar.

Above the obstruction, fluid and gas accumulate and the intestinal lumen dilates. This is exacerbated due to continuing digestion by bacteria. Peristaltic contractions increase in an attempt to move the obstruction. Later this process declines and contractions fail altogether. The area of bowel becomes oedematous, causing local and systemic fluid and electrolyte shifts. A relative hypovolaemia occurs, exacerbated by the inability to reabsorb water. Increasing distension puts pressure on the bowel wall and the blood supply is compromised – strangulation. Necrosis occurs resulting in perforation, leaking of bowel contents and subsequent peritonitis (McEntee 1999). Necrosis may also occur as a result of an ischaemic bowel due to narrowing or occlusion of the mesenteric circulation.

Clinical features

Pain

In small bowel obstruction onset of pain tends to be rapid, whereas it may be more insidious and less severe with large bowel obstruction. The character is crampy or colicky reflecting the initial excessive peristalsis. Initial pain is also likely to be central but poorly localized. Large bowel obstruction generally produces lower abdominal pain. Sharper, more severe and better localized pain suggests irritation of the peritoneum, and potentially impending perforation.

Vomiting

Profuse vomiting is a key feature of small bowel obstruction, whereas it may be absent or delayed in large bowel obstruction. Faeculent vomiting is a late feature of large bowel obstruction. Fluid lost through vomiting compounds the existing relative hypovolaemia.

Distension

Abdominal distension exacerbates the pain and may further reduce blood supply to the gut. Distension is more marked, the lower the obstruction, and is a key feature of large bowel obstruction.

Constipation

Constipation is another key feature of large bowel obstruction, but tends to be a late sign in small bowel obstruction. Constipation is considered absolute when neither faeces nor flatus is passed.

Assessment

Vital signs

The patient's observations are likely to indicate hypovolaemic shock. There may be early subtle signs such as raised respiratory rate, pulse rate and diastolic blood pressure. The pale, clammy and hypotensive patient suggests significant fluid volume deficit. The temperature may be slightly raised due to the inflammatory process.

Abdominal examination

On inspection of the abdomen, distension may be obvious, and in the thin person it may be possible to see visible peristalsis. Scars may suggest adhesions as the cause of small bowel obstruction. Auscultation often reveals high-pitched active bowel sounds reflecting the increase in peristaltic activity. Later bowel sounds become diminished or absent. Palpation is likely to illicit tenderness and guarding. It may also reveal a mass or strangulated hernia. Percussion may produce a tympanic note due to gaseous distension (Thompson 2005).

Laboratory investigations

Inflammatory markers are likely to be raised. Metabolic acidosis may be present in arterial blood gas in the shocked patient, and electrolyte levels might be deranged. Serum amylase may be slightly raised.

Radiography

Plain abdominal X-rays are standard tests in bowel obstruction. Dilated loops of bowel usually indicate the level, and potentially the cause of obstruction. Where there is still doubt contrast X-rays can be performed. If available, CT scanning may be indicated. An erect chest X-ray is mandatory if perforation is suspected, which may show air under the diaphragm.

Management

Patients with bowel obstruction are likely to require early, appropriate analgesia. Anti-emetics may be necessary, but the stomach should also be decompressed with a nasogastric (NG) tube. The patient is likely to need fluid resuscitation, and electrolyte imbalances should be corrected. Patients will be NBM and need maintenance fluids as a minimum. The patient will require close monitoring and careful re-evaluation. The surgical team may choose to manage the patient conservatively as above. Operative management is indicated immediately for evidence of strangulation, or if conservative management is unsuccessful.

Pancreatitis

Acute pancreatitis is a common surgical emergency characterized by inflammation of the pancreas.

Anatomy and physiology

The pancreas is an accessory digestive organ located in the retroperitoneum. The pancreatic duct joins the common bile duct before it reaches the duodenum. The pancreas has both endocrine and exocrine functions. The endocrine function occurs in the Islets of Langerhans, where alpha and beta cells secrete glucagon and insulin respectively. The exocrine function occurs in the acinar cells where inactive digestive enzymes are produced, such as amylase, lipase and trypsinogen. The secretion of these enzymes is stimulated by food entering the duodenum and once there, they become activated for digestion.

Aetiology and pathophysiology

Acute pancreatitis occurs as a result of many different causes, but the commonest two are gallstones and alcohol. The mechanisms by which these two factors cause pancreatitis are unclear, but certainly in gallstones, obstruction is implicated. Whatever the cause, autodigestion by prematurely activated digestive enzymes is the key pathophysiological feature. Damage to the structure of the pancreas causes inflammation and oedema. The activated digestive enzymes leak out into the area surrounding the pancreas and eventually join the systemic circulation. Local fluid losses occur, but more importantly vasodilation and increased capillary permeability cause systemic fluid shifts and a relative hypovolaemia. Other systemic effects of activated pancreatic enzymes include respiratory, renal and multi-organ failure. Necrosis of the pancreas can lead to haemorrhage, abscess formation and peritonitis. Acute pancreatitis can be mild and self-limiting or severe and life-threatening. Chronic pancreatitis is often caused by alcoholism and features frequent exacerbations due to chronic inflammatory changes (Parker 2004).

Clinical features

Pain
The pain of acute pancreatitis tends to be severe, localized to the epigastrium and radiates to the back. The pain may be described as burning, and is often worse on lying down.

Nausea and vomiting
Nausea and vomiting are common in pancreatitis, particularly if there is a recent history of alcohol consumption. Anorexia is likely as eating exacerbates the pain.

Fever
Pancreatitis is not generally an infective process, but the patient may report feeling mildly feverish due to the inflammatory process.

Assessment

There are a number of scoring criteria, which can be used to assess the severity of acute pancreatitis, such as the Ranson and Glasgow systems.

Vital signs
Accurate baseline observations and close monitoring are essential in acute pancreatitis. They can be relatively normal in mild pancreatitis, whereas there may be clear evidence of hypovolaemic shock, such as pallor, tachypnoea, tachycardia and hypotension. Low-grade pyrexia may be found.

Abdominal examination
Epigastric tenderness with guarding and rigidity are likely findings. General-ized peritonitis may be present. Rarely there may be evidence of retro-peritoneal bleeding – flank bruising (Grey Turner's sign) or peri-umbilical bruising (Cullen's sign).

Laboratory investigations
Serum amylase raised by 5–10 times is considered diagnostic for pancreatitis. Inflammatory markers are often also raised. It is important to monitor blood glucose level in pancreatitis.

Radiography

Plain abdominal X-ray may reveal a sentinel dilated loop of small bowel over the pancreas. Chest X-ray helps to exclude perforation as a differential diagnosis. CT scanning is useful to confirm the diagnosis and measure the extent of damage. An ERCP may be indicated.

Management

Treatment for acute pancreatitis is supportive. Surgery is rarely indicated. In severe presentations high concentration oxygen, aggressive fluid replacement and invasive monitoring are likely to be necessary. Opiate analgesics and anti-emetics will be required in most presentations. To rest the gut the patient should be NBM and an NG tube may be appropriate. Antibiotics may be prescribed to prevent secondary infections. Evidence of organ failure will need to be managed appropriately and the patient should be transferred to intensive care.

Peritonitis

Peritonitis is inflammation of the peritoneum and is a common cause of an 'acute abdomen'.

Anatomy and physiology

There are two layers of peritoneum in the abdominal cavity. The visceral layer covers most of the abdominal organs and is continuous with the parietal layer, which lines the abdominal wall. Between these two serous membranes is a potential space called the peritoneal cavity. This contains serous fluid, which lubricates the organs. The peritoneum is semi-permeable allowing movement of water and solutes. Some important abdominal structures are outside the peritoneal cavity in the retroperitoneum, such as the pancreas, kidneys, aorta and parts of the large bowel. The mesentery is a double layer of parietal peritoneum, which connects the visceral and parietal peritoneum. Its functions include holding the organs in place, providing a route for the vasculature and fat storage. The largest of these is the greater omentum which drapes over the small intestine like a fatty apron (Marieb and Hoehn 2007).

Aetiology and pathophysiology

Peritonitis is a secondary disease process caused by many abdominal disorders, such as perforation of the stomach, bowel or gall bladder, and penetrating abdominal trauma. Peritonitis can occur with and without infection. Initially peritonitis is localized and contained within the greater omentum and by adjoining organs. Generalized peritonitis occurs when inflammation progresses or rupture spreads contamination too far to be contained. Due to its large surface area, inflammation of the whole peritoneum results in fluid loss sufficient to cause relative hypovolaemia. This is compounded if there is a septic process superimposed (O'Kelly and Krukowski 1999).

Clinical features

Pain
Abdominal pain will be sharp and easily localized initially. With generalized peritonitis this will become diffuse, severe and exacerbated by the slightest movement.

Nausea and vomiting
Nausea and vomiting are likely to be present, if not already from the primary disorder. Any further fluid loss will exacerbate hypovolaemia.

Fever
Whether infective or not, the patient is likely to feel feverish.

Assessment

Vital signs
The patient is likely to look very unwell and have clear signs of hypovolaemic or septic shock. Respirations may be shallow to limit movement of the abdomen, resulting in poor oxygenation. The patient may also be febrile.

Abdominal examination
Findings in peritonitis include tenderness, board-like rigidity, guarding and rebound tenderness. The patient may be unable to tolerate the examination.

Laboratory investigations
The patient is likely to have raised inflammatory markers. Depending on the degree of shock there may be a metabolic acidosis on arterial blood gas analysis, and electrolyte disturbances.

Management

The priorities in managing peritonitis are resuscitation and identification of the underlying cause. Opiate analgesia, broad-spectrum antibiotics, fluid and electrolyte replacement are all indicated, along with appropriate invasive monitoring. Generalized peritonitis is an indication of laparotomy.

Renal colic

Renal or ureteral colic is a common cause of abdominal pain in the emergency department. It is more prevalent in men and recurrence is common. Renal calculi or kidney stones cause obstruction in the ureters. Pressure in the lumen causes dilation and stimulates smooth muscle contraction. If the stone doesn't move, the muscles go into spasm. The obstruction is often partial so renal failure is unlikely and the stone is usually passed spontaneously (Shokeir 2002).

Clinical features

Pain
Renal colic is one of the most intense forms of pain. As the name suggests, pain is colicky in nature and comes in waves. Pain is in the flank or loin and may radiate to the back, groin or genitals – loin to groin pain. The patient often writhes in pain and is unable to find a comfortable position. The pain may mimic appendicitis on the right side.

Nausea and vomiting
Pain-induced vomiting is common in renal colic.

Haematuria
Microscopic haematuria is a key diagnostic factor in renal colic.

Assessment

Vital signs
The patient is likely to be tachycardic due to the pain. It may be impossible to take full observations until the patient has been given pain relief. The patient may be pale and diaphoretic.

Urinalysis
It is important to gain a urine sample as soon as possible, but this also may be difficult due to pain. Blood is found on urinalysis.

Laboratory investigations
Routine blood tests should be performed as a baseline, to assess renal function and exclude other diagnoses.

Radiography

The traditional investigation of choice for renal colic was intravenous urography or pyelography (IVU or IVP), but this requires IV contrast and is time-consuming. Helical CT scan is now the gold standard investigation for renal colic, as it is rapid, accurate and will identify other diagnoses (Teichman 2004). Ripolles et al. (2004) found CT more accurate than combined plain X-ray and ultrasound scan, but concluded that this is a practical alternative.

Management

Early pain relief is the main priority in renal colic. It responds well to non-steroidal anti-inflammatory drugs (NSAID), such as diclofenac. NSAIDs reduce inflammation and inhibit ureteric smooth muscle contraction. This can be given rectally if the patient is vomiting. Caution should be taken in patients with existing renal disease and a history of GI bleeding. Opiates are the second-line analgesics in renal colic. Anti-emetics can be given if the patient is vomiting. Traditionally patients have been encouraged to increase fluid intake (oral or IV) to flush the stones out, however, Worster and Richards (2005) found that there is little evidence to support this. Stones, which do not pass spontaneously, may be removed by lithotripsy, ureteroscopy or surgery (Anagnostou and Tolley 2004).

Abdominal aortic aneurysm (AAA)

Scenario 7.2 Abdominal aortic aneurysm
A 69-year-old man is brought in by ambulance after collapsing at home. His wife states that he had been complaining of abdominal pain beforehand. He has a history of ischaemic heart disease and hypertension. On arrival his respiratory rate is 27, pulse 112bpm and blood pressure is 92/64 mmHg.

D *Data* **(scientific facts):** the nurse will need to assess this patient in a resuscitation area and alert senior colleagues. The patient will require continuous monitoring, bilateral blood pressures and an urgent ECG. The vital signs suggest decompensated shock, but other data should be sought, such as evidence of pallor. The history suggests AAA, but cardiac causes will need to be excluded. Further data will include physical examination, baseline blood tests and cardiac enzymes.

E *Emotions* **(intuition):** the assessor's gut reaction is AAA, however, the priorities for this critically ill patient is an ABCDE approach and initial stabilization. Previous experience of AAA should alert the nurse to the severity of the situation.

A *Advantages*: a team approach to assessment and stabilization of this patient will expedite diagnosis and a definitive management plan. When diagnosis of AAA is made, permissive hypotension, rather than aggressive fluid management is indicated.

D *Disadvantages* (**differential diagnosis**): other causes of this presentation include myocardial infarction and an early ECG will rule this in or out and guide alternative therapy.

Aetiology and pathophysiology

A dissecting or ruptured aortic aneurysm can cause patients to present to the emergency department with an 'acute abdomen' or collapse.

The aorta is the main artery taking blood from the heart to the systemic circulation. The descending aorta passes posteriorly through the thoracic and abdominal cavities. Arteries are composed of three layers: the tunica intima on the inside, the muscular tunica media in the middle and the tunica adventitia on the outside. An aneurysm is a weakening and subsequent dilatation of a blood vessel. This is often due to atherosclerosis and is commonest in the aorta. Blood flow may cause the vessel to bulge or it may separate the layers for some distance. This is called a dissecting aneurysm and can affect other organs such as the kidneys. If an aneurysm ruptures, blood loss into the retroperitoneum may be gradual, but it is often catastrophic and fatal. AAA is commonest in elderly patients with a history of cardiovascular disease.

Clinical features

Pain
Pain from a dissecting AAA is classically described as a sudden tearing or ripping pain in the central abdomen or chest, and radiates through to the back or to the groin. There may be little or no pain in the early stages allowing the AAA to go undetected. Patients may also just present with back pain.

Collapse
Sudden rupture and blood loss are likely to result in collapse, and AAA should be a differential diagnosis for all collapsed and shocked elderly patients, until proven otherwise.

Dizziness
Whether the patient has collapsed or not they are likely to feel faint or dizzy if rupture or dissection is present.

Nausea and vomiting
Hypovolaemic or pain-induced nausea and vomiting are not uncommon in AAA.

Assessment

Vital signs

The hypovolaemic patient will show clear signs of shock. There may also be a reduced level of consciousness. There is often a significant difference in blood pressure between the right and left arm. An ECG should be taken immediately.

Abdominal examination

A tender, pulsatile mass is found on palpation in most patients with AAA. In some cases pulsations are visible above the umbilicus. Altered distal blood supply can manifest as weak or absent femoral pulses and mottled skin.

Laboratory investigations

Diagnosis of AAA is a clinical one, but baseline blood tests are essential. Haemoglobin will be normal in the acute phase unless there is pre-existing anaemia. Amylase and cardiac enzymes are useful in ruling out other diagnoses and blood should be urgently cross-matched.

Radiography

Chest X-ray may show a widened mediastinum. AAA is visible on ultrasound, which can be performed at the bedside. CT scan and angiography should only be performed on stable patients.

Management

Patients with suspected AAA require close monitoring in a resuscitation area. Early surgical review is vital, and once a diagnosis is reached, urgent preparations should be made for theatre. Opiate analgesia will be required, high concentration oxygen and early IV access are essential, but permissive hypotension rather than aggressive fluid resuscitation is indicated. Fluids may exacerbate bleeding so low blood pressure is accepted. The priority is rapid, definitive treatment. Surgery includes open or endovascular repair, but the mortality is still 60–80 per cent following AAA rupture (Ohki and Veith 2004).

Conclusion

A wide variety of acute surgical emergencies prompt patients to attend emergency departments. The commonest presenting complaint is abdominal pain, but patients also present with a range of other symptoms. Accurate history and examination provide much of the information needed to reach a diagnosis. Emergency practitioners have a key role in data collection, providing symptom relief and expediting definitive management.

8   Head injuries

Cliff Evans

Introduction

All frontline or acute healthcare professionals require the ability to make a quick and efficient assessment of individuals who have sustained either an injury to their head or have the potential to acquire a loss of cerebral function. The ability to appropriately assess focuses on the clinician understanding the basic form and function of the brain and applying a structured approach to their delivery of care. This chapter centres on facilitating clinicians to gain those skills and apply a solid evidence base to their clinical practice.

The brain

The human psyche still remains a mystery, as does its controlling organ: the brain is responsible for interpreting electrical impulses into mental phenomena, conscious thought and the vital physiological role it plays in controlling involuntary mechanisms and maintaining homeostasis.

This vital component to both mental and physical function is well protected with internal regulatory mechanisms geared at self-preservation and strong physical protection in the form of bone and surrounding membranes.

It takes a considerable force or impact to penetrate these protective barriers and directly traumatize the brain. Despite this, there are several ways in which the brain is vulnerable to damage, any of which can result in a traumatic brain injury (TBI).

Definition and prevalence

A head injury is defined as any trauma to the head other than superficial injuries to the face (NICE 2003). Head trauma refers to direct or indirect impact to the head that results in some degree of actual brain damage/injury referred to as a TBI (Traumatic Brain Injury).

Within the UK it is estimated that around 700,000 individuals attend hospital with varying degrees of head injury every year, 40–50 per cent of whom are under 16 (NICE 2003). Alcohol is associated with around 50 per cent of the adult attendances. Increasing age is associated with an increased risk of intracranial complications and a poorer prognosis.

Head injuries make up around 1 per cent of all deaths, the most susceptible age range being between 5 and 35 years old where TBI accounts for around 20 per cent of all deaths.

The three main causes of head injuries are falls, assaults and road traffic accidents (RTA). Head injuries from RTAs alone are responsible for in excess of 2500 deaths each year in the UK. In the USA around 250,000 individuals per annum are hospitalized with head injuries with a mortality rate exceeding 50,000 (Langlois et al. 2004).

The continuum of TBI is best viewed as a two-part process. First, the initial insult; when a patient presents for emergency treatment following a head injury, the primary damage has already taken place, therefore the focus of treatment centres on managing the primary injury and preventing secondary injury development. Secondary brain injury is mostly preventable: by closely monitoring the patient for the signs and symptoms associated with physical deterioration or further brain injury, the clinician can reduce both morbidity and mortality rates.

Patients will be assessed using the ABCDE approach to establish the actual level of injury present. This should be undertaken in combination with the gathering of a succinct picture of the events preceding the injury; this enables the clinician to formulate a risk assessment on the potential for secondary brain damage (Box 8.1).

In 2003, the National Institute for Health and Clinical Excellence (NICE) released guidelines outlining a clinical standard for patients experiencing a head injury. Empirically these guidelines have already had a significant impact on clinical practice. Subjective individual practice has been replaced by a constructive patient-centred approach that is easy to follow, professionally empowering and most importantly, critical for the patient's prognosis. The guidelines have resulted in a lower threshold for, and easier access to, definitive scanning tests such as computerized tomography (CT).

For clinicians to be in a position to make sound clinical judgements on either the assessment, risk potential or treatment of the head-injured patient, they require a sound foundational knowledge of the relevant anatomy of the head and both the basic physiology, and pathophysiology associated with TBI. This will enable the clinician to construct a detailed mental picture containing the mechanism of injury, the actual and potential injuries and the instigation of a structured plan of treatment.

Box 8.1	Risk factors synonymous with traumatic brain injury

- GCS less than 15 at any time since injury.
- Loss of consciousness as a result of the injury.
- Focal neurological deficit since the injury (decreased comprehension, sensation or ability to talk; loss of balance; visual disturbances).
- Suspicion of a skull fracture (otorrhoea/rhinorrhoea, ecchymosis without trauma to the eyes or ears, acute deafness, mechanism of injury or clinical signs indicating potential for penetrating injury).
- Amnesia prior to or post-injury.
- Persistent headache post-injury.
- Clinical judgement should be used regarding episodes of vomiting post-injury.
- Seizure post-injury.
- Previous cranial neurosurgical interventions.
- A high-energy/impact head injury (pedestrian struck by motor vehicle, occupant ejected from motor vehicle, a fall from a height of greater than one metre or more than five stairs, diving accident, high-speed motor vehicle collision, rollover motor accident, or other high energy mechanism).
- A lower threshold for height of falls should be used when dealing with infants and young children.
- Patient history of bleeding, clotting disorders, or current anti-coagulant therapy.
- Drug or alcohol intoxication; age greater than or equal to 65 years; suspicion of non-accidental injury.

Source: Based on NICE (2003) guidelines

Anatomy and physiology

The head or skull is a well-fortified solidly formed protective barrier for the controlling mechanism of the human body. The skull is covered in both skin in the form of the scalp and muscle, which protect the area and allow for movement of the facial muscles. The scalp is spread very thinly across the skull and has an excellent blood supply hence a laceration here will result in a large superficial amount of bleeding.

The skull is classically described in two distinct parts, first, the cranium, consisting of eight bones, forming a vault, which contains the brain and, second, the face, comprising 14 bones which culminate to form the mandible, protect the facial cavities and provide an attachment point for the complex musculature of the face. There are several small openings into the cranium allowing the passage of blood vessels and nerves. The major inlet and outlet is the foramen magnum at the base of the skull, which allows passage of the spinal cord.

The major bones of the skull are fixed, with dense connective tissue and cartilage adding strength to the structure. In contrast, the mandible facilitates the passage of food and is therefore a highly movable joint. As with all movable or pivotal joints, the mandible is at serious risk of fracture or dislocation when injured.

Three closely adjacent layers surround the brain and its extension: the spinal cord the dura, arachnoid and pia mater (Figure 8.1).

The dura mater is the outermost layer, which replaces the periosteum on the inner surface of the skull; it directly surrounds the brain and at various suture points suspends the brain within the skull. In addition it provides further protection. The potential spaces between the dural layer and the skull are referred to as the epidural or extradural spaces. Deoxygenated blood drains into sinuses between these layers flowing toward the jugular veins. The second layer is the arachnoid mater, which again is separated from the dural layer by a potential space: the subdural space. The arachnoid mater is the first layer to mix with the cerebral spinal fluid for which it provides the medium for reabsorption.

The arachnoid and innermost layer, the pia mater, are separated by the subarachnoid space, rich in cerebrospinal fluid. The pia mater is the layer that

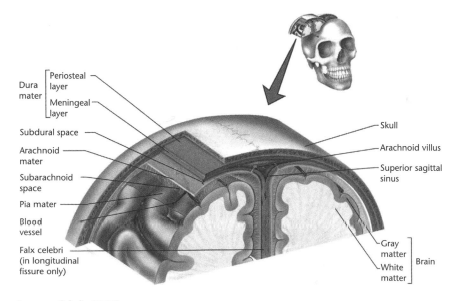

Source: Saladin (2005)

Figure 8.1 The meninges

merges with the brain and contains a rich supply of blood vessels. These three layers, collectively called the meninges, provide protection and assist in the maintenance of homeostasis.

Anatomically the brain is composed of several lobes that combine to form the central controlling mechanism of the human body. The key areas are as follows:

- The cerebrum, which contains the right and left hemispheres.
- The hemispheres receive sensory information and control motor function on the opposite side of the body, processing conscious thought and reasoning skills (Figure 8.2).

Box 8.2 Major areas involved in head injuries

- Scalp
- Skull injuries (open or closed); protective membranes – meninges (dura, arachnoid and pia mater)
- Meningeal/potential spaces epidural/subdural/subarachnoid
- Meningeal/cerebral arteries
- Cerebral spinal fluid (CSF) pathways
- Lobes of the brain
- Brain stem and associated control centres
- Foramen magnum

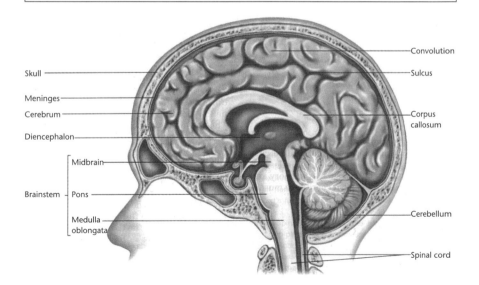

Source: Shire et al. (2004) (Reproduced with the permission of the McGraw-Hill companies)

Figure 8.2 The major portions of the brain

- The frontal lobes are considered to be the central point of intelligence and the site of advanced development.
- The parietal lobes receive sensory information including the senses of temperature, pain, touch and pressure; they also play a role in the acquisition of memory.
- The occipital lobes contain the visual cortex and interpret impulses as visual information.
- The temporal lobes consist of areas of sensory information including the auditory cortex.
- The diencephalon lies deep within the cerebrum and consists of two vital control centres: the hypothalamus and the thalamus. The hypothalamus lies at the base of the brain and controls autonomic nervous system activity, in combination with the lobes of the pituitary gland; it regulates hormonal influence over the involuntary actions within the body maintaining homeostasis (Chapter 2).
- The thalamus is a relay point, mainly for sensory information travelling between the area of interpretation and the cerebral cortex.
- The brainstem is composed of the medulla, the pons and the midbrain (Figure 8.3). The midbrain is commonly referred to as a relay station, and plays several important roles including the regulation of

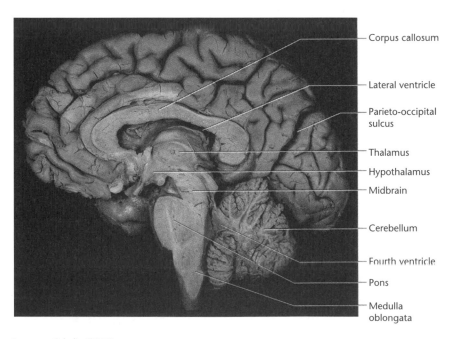

Corpus callosum

Lateral ventricle

Parieto-occipital sulcus

Thalamus

Hypothalamus

Midbrain

Cerebellum

Fourth ventricle

Pons

Medulla oblongata

Source: Saladin (2005)

Figure 8.3 The brain

eye movement. It connects with the basal ganglia and extrapyramidal tracts, which are involved in muscle contraction. The midbrain also contains part of the reticular activating system (RAS) responsible for determining the sleep/wake cycle.

- The cerebellum connects to several other areas of the brain including the medulla oblongata. Although involved in many higher activities, the cerebellum is best known for its function in coordinating fine motor movement and standing and walking.
- The medulla oblongata links the brain and spinal cord; it is within the medulla that tracts or pathways from the left side of the brain decussate (cross over) to the opposite side of the spinal cord. The physical result of this cross-over is that information from one side of the body is passed over to the opposite side of the brain, thereby making the right side of the brain responsible for the left side of the body. The medulla oblongata works closely with the hypothalamus to regulate the vital control centres of respiratory, cardiac and vaso-motor function.

Damage will directly compromise the affected areas' functional ability resulting in the termination of neural messages. Damage can be localized or diffuse, associated with or without cerebral oedema or haemorrhage.

Primary damage and directional forces

Primary damage is a direct outcome of the initial impact and can include many injuries that will lead to a secondary injury developing (Box 8.3). When a force is applied to the head, a TBI can result, and damage arises from one or a combination of the following:

- Structural characteristics of the skull and its contents
- The direction of the force
- The amount of kinetic energy applied to the skull and its contents.

The combination of the rigidity of the skull and the internal contours places the soft brain tissue at great risk of bruising and haematoma formation when a force is applied to the skull. Contusions are the most common manifestation of brain injury and usually occur at two sights. The first occurs directly at the impact point; referred to as a coup contusion, the second injury arises as the force of impact drives the brain backwards, the opposite area of brain tissue rebounds off of the skull, referred to as a contrecoup contusion. The attachment points between the dura mater and the lower layers can rip, resulting in bleeding. Most of the energy of impact from a

---

Box 8.3 Primary damage

Lacerations – cuts and tears, more likely to occur in frontal or temporal lobes. The frontal area of the skull has far better protection than the temporal region, which is thinner and has superficial blood vessels running beneath it.

Contusions – bruising, areas of bruising where tissue changes, depending on the amount of local damage may result in cellular death.

Skull fractures – depending on type of fracture and affected area, may result in secondary damage to underlying structures.

Diffuse axonal injury (DAI) – axons (the communication cords between cells) have been ripped apart. Associated damage can be very diffuse and widespread.

Haemorrhage – vessel or tissues are ripped during injury, resulting in bleeding.

---

small hard object tends to dissipate at the impact site, leading to a coup contusion, impact from a larger object causes less injury at the impact site since the energy is dissipated leading to a contrecoup contusion. It is therefore easy to see how a combination of vascular and tissue damage leads to cerebral contusion.

Depending on the direction and energy applied at the time of initial impact, a shearing force can occur to the contents of the skull, this usually involves rapid movement. The prime instigator leading to rapid and vigorous movements of the head are usually the consequences of RTAs. The rapid acceleration and deceleration of the head and neck can result in dire consequences; these shearing forces cause different areas of the brain to move relative to one another. It is this motion that produces the stretching and tearing of axons, whose function is normally to conduct or transmit electrical messages; when disrupted, this culminates in diffuse axonal injuries that interrupt the reticular activating system producing a loss of consciousness.

Concussion (jolting of the brain) has various classifications beginning with mild, in which consciousness is preserved and characterized by a temporary neurological dysfunction, or disorientation. In classic cerebral concussion the brain may suffer a brief interruption to the reticular activating system (RAS), which causes a short period of unconsciousness and possibly amnesia. If the injury affects many neurons and their axons, the result can be prolonged post-traumatic coma accompanied with autonomic nervous system dysfunction referred to as a diffuse axonal injury (DAI).

Secondary damage

Secondary damage is usually due to hypoxic changes related to hypovolaemia or an increased intracranial pressure either, and can result in the impairment of cerebral oxygen delivery (Box 8.4).

Box 8.4 Secondary damage

Haematoma – occurs after bleeding, puts pressure on the brain and can displace the brain from its normal position.
Cerebral oedema – resulting damage dependent on location and severity.
Hypoxic-ischaemic damage – even if the brain gets blood, it still doesn't receive enough oxygen. This will cause localized damage or death. Causes include chest wall instability, damage to the cardiac/respiratory/vasomotor centres.
Seizures – over-excitation of brain activity. Results in cerebral oedema, hypoxia and increased metabolic demand.

Types of head injury

Head injuries can be classified in various ways; for the purpose of a succinct overview the following section will categorize head injuries as either external or internal:

- External (usually involving the scalp) – Due to the rich blood supply, these injuries have the potential to bleed profusely when the skin or muscle of the head is lacerated or punctured. If the injury fails to lacerate the scalp but damages vessels underlying the scalp, the resulting bleeding or swelling produces the classic 'goose egg' appearance commonly seen in children; these types of superficial injury are usually self-limiting.
- Internal (involving the skull, the meningeal layers and their potential spaces, major blood vessels or parts of the brain) – The skull forms a rigid and fixed closed box, commonly referred to as a vault. The clinical implication of which is that if bleeding or swelling occurs within the skull, a raised pressure will ensue (due to the inability of the skull to expand), this is referred to as an increased intracranial pressure (ICP). The pressure within the skull is created by its components, i.e., the brain, cerebral spinal fluid (CSF) and blood. CSF is continuously secreted and reabsorbed into the blood plasma so that a state of internal equilibrium can be maintained. A head injury may result in an increase in volume by disrupting the reabsorption, increasing the secretion; alternatively tissue and vessel damage may result in a disruption of the circulatory cycle resulting in the continual secretion of CSF and an ever-increasing internal pressure. The term cerebral oedema refers to an increased intracranial fluid volume.

Skull fracture

The skull bones can be fractured in exactly the same way as other bones, although to obtain a significant brain injury does not necessitate a fractured skull. There is, however, a 12-fold increased risk of TBI in a patient with a fractured skull; this is because the skull will not absorb the entire force of impact. The force or kinetic energy necessary to damage the skull will continue to dissipate directly through the meninges and into the brain (NICE 2003). Clinically a skull fracture is of little importance, hence the demise of routine skull X-rays. The advent and liberal use of CT imagery reveal both bone abnormalities and damage to the underlying structures. The identification of the area affected is important as certain areas are anatomically at greater risk than others. Impact to the frontoparietal region may result in partial or complete rupture of the superficial lying middle meningeal artery. Anatomically this artery lies between the skull and the dura, when damaged, the resulting bleeding expands to fill the potential space between the dura mater and the skull. The bleeding forms an extradural or epidural haematoma; this expanding haematoma formation exerts increasing pressure within the skull and onto sensitive areas of the brain. The resulting alterations to both sensory and motor activity, in addition to the alterations to vital signs and pupillary size and reactivity, reveal a potential myriad of clinical signs and symptoms. Eventually this process can result in the sensitive brain tissue being compressed or expanding, depending on the origin of the bleeding. Either way, neural functioning will be affected, and may result in neural loss and the possibility of brain tissue being forced against or through the tentorial notch/foramen magnum, which poses the only escape route. This can result in brainstem herniation/coning and imminent death as the vital centres within the brainstem are literally compressed through the hole.

The assessment

In the UK, national guidelines identify the minimum assessment criteria at the triage stage of acute presentations (NICE 2003). These guidelines minimize the chance of subjective and misjudged practice compromising a patient's care.

The focal point of assessing an individual with a head injury is to identify the presence of a clinically important brain injury, and the risk potential for secondary damage development. A suitably qualified member of staff must assess all patients presenting to the emergency department with a head injury within 15 minutes of arrival. If a decreased level of consciousness is identified, immediate in-depth assessment is indicated (NICE 2003). The initial assessment consists of identifying the mechanism of injury which may also identify a risk to the cervical spine, recording baseline physiological findings, i.e., respiratory rate, pulse and blood pressure, pupillary response and an assessment of the patient's Glasgow coma score (GCS) which should follow the quick and easy to utilize AVPU score (Chapter 2).

The assessment and need for intervention should be guided primarily by the use of the GCS in combination with the pupillary response and motor power (NICE 2003). It is essential, therefore, that all clinicians gain extensive experience of its clinical application. The GCS is a subjective tool and is not therefore, foolproof, it should be used in conjunction with an overview of the patient's vital signs and the presenting mechanism of injury, as this will provide minimal variation and individual subjectivity in the initial and ongoing clinical assessment of neurological impairment (Box 8.5 provides an overview).

Box 8.5 Recording a Glasgow coma scale

E Eye response: when assessing for eye response, ask yourself, does the patient appear aware of their surroundings and do they acknowledge your presence when you enter their eye line? Does it take a verbal stimulus to arouse their attention? If needed, a painful stimulus can be achieved by using your thumb and index finger to squeeze the patient's trapezius muscle, but an alternative is to apply pressure to the groove along the supraorbital margin just above the eyelid (beware of co-existing facial trauma). These are the recommended stimuli as peripheral pathways such as the nail beds may be compromised.

V Verbal response: does the patient know who and where they are? Time and place: does the patient know what year and month/season they are in, and why they are here? (Who? Where? Why?) Has the patient the ability to conduct a conversation but fails to answer correctly (confused)? The patient may fail to connect words and speech is random or unorganized (inappropriate words). Incomprehensible sounds refer to noises not speech.

M Motor response: When a patient responds appropriately to a physical request, it demonstrates their ability to act on interpreted data but this ability may be compromised by acute or chronic physical disabilities. Localizing to pain requires the patient to coordinate motor activity by attempting to remove the stimulus. A decorticate or spastic flexion response indicates an interruption of the neural pathways. A decerebrate or extension of a limb away from the stimulus has a poor prognosis.

Neurological observations are a vital part of the care continuum for patients with a possible head injury, therefore they must be recorded, this includes waking the patient, as a sleeping patient could indicate a comatose patient.

The GCS consists of three components that combine to reveal an in-depth picture of the individual's level of conscious, in other words, they show the effectiveness or ease with which the individual is stimulated (sense/arousal), interprets a stimulus or evidences their cognitive ability (reasoning skills) and conveys a response (motor function) appropriately (Table 8.1).

The GCS is not foolproof: many individual or combined factors can affect the reliability of the scores, these are summarized in Box 8.6. The clinician should also consider the possibility of chronic sensual impairments such as deafness when recording data.

Table 8.1 The Glasgow coma scale

Assessment area	Score
Eye opening (E):	
Spontaneous	4
To speech	3
To pain	2
None	1
Verbal response (V):	
Orientated	5
Confused conversation	4
Inappropriate words	3
Incomprehensible sounds	2
None	1
Best motor response (M):	
Obeys commands	6
Localizes to pain	5
Normal flexion (withdrawal)	4
Abnormal flexion (decorticate)	3
Extension (decerebrate)	2
No response (flaccid)	1

Source: Based on the scale developed by Teasdale and Jennett (1974)

NICE (2003) recommends that the score for each of the three sections is individually recorded and conveyed professionally.

The underpinning rationale to current clinical practice is focused on identifying risk and instigating early imaging, rather than admission and

---

Box 8.6 Compromising factors

The following notations can be inserted into the relevant GCS box as the data may be compromised:

\# Fracture or pathology limiting movement
C   Used to denote a closed eye: gross swelling or a prosthetic eye
D   Used if a patient is unable to communicate in an effective manner due to dysphasia
P   Pharmacological intervention may hinder clinical assessment (anaesthetics)
T   The patient has had a intervention that interferes with speech (intubation)

observation. This is seen to reduce the detection time for life-threatening complications and results in better outcomes (NICE 2003). Patients found to be at increased risk of brain injury at triage should be fully assessed within 10 minutes by an appropriately trained member of staff; this assessment must include the clinician deciding whether or not the patient requires a CT scan of the head or cervical spine. The Canadian CT-head rules form the rationale and evidence base for clinical decision-making (Box 8.7)

To scan or not to scan

Computerized tomography (CT) is seen to be the gold standard diagnostic test when presented with a patient experiencing a potential brain injury. NICE (2003) recommend that all clinicians involved in the assessment of those experiencing a head injury should be able to negate or consolidate the presence or absence of the risk factors used in the Canadian CT-head and cervical spine rules, thereby rationalizing their practice. These factors are identified in Box 8.7.

> **Scenario 8.1**   Epidural bleed
>
> Saeed Patel, a 19-year-old male, attends following an assault. He states some local gang members attacked him around one hour ago, after he left an infamous local nightclub. He was knocked to the floor and is unsure if he lost consciousness, there were no witnesses.
>
> His respiratory rate is 23 and regular. There are no signs of central or peripheral cyanosis. His radial pulse is strong, regular and recorded as 92 bpm, CRT is within two seconds. The initial blood pressure is recorded as 140/87. Mr Patel appears agitated, and states he will wait no longer than 30 minutes to be seen. He appears pale, has dried blood around his nose and several minor abrasions and lacerations to his face and hands. His shirt has vomit stains and dried blood on it. His GCS is recorded as 15/15 although his speech is slurred and he is hard to understand at times.
>
> His pupils are equal and reactive to light and recorded as 4mm. He smells heavily of alcohol, and states he has had a 'few' and that the left side of his head hurts. He has no relevant medical history.
>
> Fifteen minutes later his GCS is recorded as E3 V4 M5 = 12/15.

D *Data* (scientific facts): Mr Patel is able to convey the history to his presentation despite his slurred speech, and has his initial GCS recorded as 15. Initially he demonstrates physical signs associated with sympathetic nervous system activation. These include tachypnoea, and an elevation to his heart rate and

---

Box 8.7 To scan or not to scan

Are any of the following present?

- GCS <13 at any point since the incident
- GCS <13/14 two hours post injury
- Focal neurological deficit
- Suspected open or depressed skull fracture
- Any clinical signs of basal skull fracture?
- Post-traumatic seizure
- Vomiting episodes (clinical judgement should be used on aetiology)

Yes   No
↓

Any loss of consciousness or amnesia post-incident?

Yes   No
↓

Are any of the following present?

- Age > 65
- Coagulopathy (warfarin therapy, clotting disorders)

Yes   No
↓

Are any of the following present?

- Dangerous mechanism of injury
- Amnesia of greater than 30 mins for events before incident

Yes   No
↓

| Request CT imaging of the head immediately – imaging to be done within one hour of request | Request CT imaging of the head immediately – scanning to be carried out within 8 hours of the injury – or immediately if they present > 8 hours of injury | No test required |

(Based on NICE (2003) guidelines)

blood pressure. This response could be due to pain, psychological trauma or anxiety. The respiratory rate is raised and following an assault a pneumothorax should always be negated. He demonstrates bi-lateral air entry and has no difficulty in breathing. An oxygen saturation level should be recorded in all patients exhibiting tachypnoea to establish a baseline. Mr Patel's radial pulse is strong and regular, in conjunction with the normal CRT, physiological shock is negated at this time, although he should be fully exposed to reveal unseen areas such as the abdomen and back which may reveal insidious signs. His blood pressure is slightly raised and should be reviewed in relation to other vital signs every 15–30 minutes. His blood sugar should be monitored in case of alcohol-induced hypoglycaemia. Initially Mr Patel does not require a CT scan according to the NICE (2003) guidelines; although he does demonstrate risk factors for a TBI, these include the possibility of a loss of consciousness, slurred speech, at least one episode of vomiting and alcohol ingestion.

E *Emotions* (**intuition**): the scenario of Mr Patel's presentation will be familiar to all emergency care staff. A patient presents after an assault. Commonly the first question the patient asks is how long 'it' is going to take. If the clinician fails to respond professionally, this encounter can proceed with the potential for a poor patient/practitioner relationship, disruption to the department or even violence. At the initial assessment it should be made clear to the patient that the practitioner is acting in their best interests and that, due to the nature of their injury, regular neurological observations will need to be undertaken over the next few hours. When the potential seriousness of their predicament is professionally expressed to the patient, they take it seriously, and the practitioner does not become part of the negative picture the patient may currently have with regard to others.

The experienced clinician may consider that his full assessment should take place within 10 minutes, although when adhering strictly to the guidelines, this is not the case. He should therefore be placed in an area with suction and oxygen in case of sudden deterioration or vomiting, and regular, neurological observations undertaken according to the national guidelines (Box 8.8).

A *Advantages*: intoxicated patients present many problems for front-line practitioners: unruly behaviour, confrontation and the potential for a misdiagnosis are high. It is therefore imperative to apply a structured and professional approach to their care.

The lack of a reliable witness to the preceding events means the presentation should be taken seriously as the patient may have been knocked unconscious. Initially oxygen therapy is unnecessary although as with his or her other vital signs, his or her respiratory rate should be regularly monitored. Intravenous cannulation and bloods are unnecessary although many emergency departments may have a protocol on administering fluids to

> **Box 8.8** Recording of vital signs in a patient experiencing a head injury
>
> - Observations should be recorded on a half-hourly basis until the GCS is 15
> - Half-hourly for two hours > if stable continue to ↓
> - One hourly for four hours > if stable continue to ↓
> - Two hourly thereafter.
>
> This is a progressive scale and patients should not progress unless their clinical signs indicate so. Any sign of neurological deterioration should instigate immediate re-assessment by the supervising team and the patient should revert to half-hourly observations and follow the original plan of care, this includes:
>
> - The development or increasing agitation or abnormal behaviour
> - A sustained drop of one point in the GCS for 30 minutes
> - A drop in GCS greater than two points regardless of duration
> - Severe or increasing headache or persistent vomiting
> - The development of any neurological signs including: pupil inequality, asymmetric movements
> - Any physical changes putting the patient at increased risk, i.e., seizures.

potentially intoxicated attendees. Regular blood glucose levels should be obtained, as hypoglycaemia secondary to alcohol intoxication is a common finding (McQuillan et al. 2002). The plan of care for Mr Patel centres on close, neurological observation in case of sudden deterioration and the prevention of secondary brain damage (Figure 8.4).

D *Disadvantages* (**differential diagnosis**): when faced with a patient presenting in a stable condition, but with risk factors for serious illness and a significant

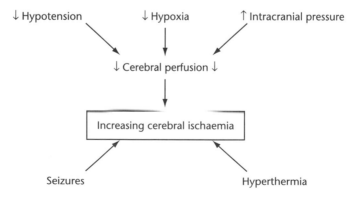

Figure 8.4 Summary of secondary damage development

presenting history, the practitioner must proceed with caution when making a working diagnosis.

Slurred speech and agitated behaviour are frequently attributed to alcohol intoxication; this should only be the case when a TBI has fully been negated, as slurred speech or dysphasia can have serious implications including damage to the cerebellum or brainstem. The speech centre of the brain is usually located on the left side even when the individual is left-handed. If this area has been affected, the patient may not be able to form proper words, or recall a particular word/object. For normal speech to occur, the muscles of the tongue, throat and larynx must work together, therefore, many factors can affect the individual's ability to speak clearly.

Mr Patel has been assaulted and therefore a full assessment including exposure of areas of potential bleeding is advised. Abdominal or flank tenderness are potential indicators of a traumatic injury. His ribs should be felt for injury potential and his extremities observed for minor injuries (Chapter 5).

Sudden deterioration

Mr Patel's GCS suddenly deteriorates: he is reassessed using the ABCDE approach.

A   The patency of his airway will be re-assessed, he is still able to talk although he is now confused to his surroundings and to what is happening.

B   His respiratory rate is recorded as 10 with bilateral chest expansion and no difficulties noted, oxygen saturation is 98 per cent on air; high-flow oxygen is commenced.

C   The radial pulse is strong regular and 52bpm, CRT remains within two seconds. Blood pressure is recorded as 170/98.

D   GCS: E3 V4 M5 = 12/15. The pupils are re-examined and a difference noted. Left pupil 4mm and reactive to light. Right pupil 6mm and non-reactive.

E   Tympanic temperature 37.9. No physical signs of bleeding, bruising or fluid loss noted.

In Mr Patel's scenario the risk potential was real and he has developed the physical manifestation of a TBI. This is clearly demonstrated in the vital signs as bradycardia, bradypnoea and hypertension (referred to as Cushing's triad). The potential of an intracranial bleed is high and a CT scan is immediately indicated. He will require specialist assistance, despite his GCS currently indicating a moderate head injury (Table 8.2), the potential for further deterioration is high and an anaesthetist should be requested. The results of the CT scan will reveal an epidural bleed, thereby necessitating referral and assessment by a neurosurgeon.

Table 8.2 Classification of head injury (A GCS of 8 or less has become the accepted definition of coma)

Damage	Glasgow coma score	Attendees (%)
Mild	GCS 14–15	90
Moderate	GCS 9–13	5
Severe	GCS 3–8	5

Based on the NICE (2003) guidelines

Patients presenting with epidural bleeds usually have a recent history of head injury with or without a loss of consciousness, typically within a couple of hours the patient will experience a decrease in their level of consciousness and potentially a paralysis affecting one side of their body due to the expanding haematoma compressing one side of the brain. This will need surgical evacuation as soon as possible, epidural bleeds have a mortality rate of between 25–50 per cent, and subdural bleeds a mortality rate of 70 per cent (NICE 2003).

There is little evidence to support any other preliminary aggressive therapies other than the definitive clot removal. Secondary injury prevention is paramount, maximal oxygenation; an adequate mean arterial pressure (Chapter 2) and a normative temperature are essential. This is vital as for every 1°C rise in body temperature there is approximately a 10 per cent elevation in cerebral oxygen consumption. The specialist centres protocol should be followed as regards the administration of osmotic diuretics or other therapies directed at reducing ICP in the interim period.

Head injury and pupillary changes

Pupillary changes are usually a late sign of head injury although sluggishly reacting pupils can manifest early into the presentation and are a sinister warning sign (American College of Surgeons 2004). Pupillary response should be evaluated in conjunction with the presenting history and vital sign analysis. If possible, ascertain any chronic irregularities to the patient's pupils, i.e., cataract formation, blindness or a prosthetic eye. When pressure increases within the cranium, or is directed against a particular area of the brain, the result can be that areas toward the rear of the brain are stretched or squeezed against the tentorial notch or foramen magnum as this presents the only escape valve. The brain stem can become compressed or herniate resulting in damage to its blood supply and potential haemorrhage in the midbrain and pons, which affects the RAS, causing rapidly deepening coma. The third cranial nerve (oculomotor) passes close to the opening and is displaced or

---

Box 8.9 Pupillary measurement

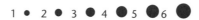

1 • 2 ● 3 ● 4 ● 5 ● 6 ●

Before testing the pupillary light reflex, identify the size, shape, and symmetry of the patient's pupils.

Normal pupil size is 2 to 5mm. Ask the patient to look straight ahead. The light should be brought into the line of the sight on a horizontal plan and briefly pointed at the pupil, the assessor should note if constriction of the pupil takes place and if it is brisk (= +), sluggish (Sl) or if there is no reaction (= –).

---

stretched by tentorial herniation. Both parasympathetic and sympathetic fibres innervate the eye to control pupil size. Parasympathetic influence via the oculomotor nerve cause pupillary constriction, when the midbrain or oculomotor nerve are compressed, the parasympathetic innervation is blocked and the sympathetic fibres dominate, causing mydriasis (dilation). Dilation of the pupils can also be achieved by the use of Benzodiazepines and drugs that affect the ANS such as atropine and adrenaline. Miosis (constriction) of intracranial origin is due to pontine or diencephalic dysfunction; this can also be instigated by drugs such as opioids. The points for sympathetic innervation are via the hypothalamus, the Pons, and the cervical ganglion, pontine pupils are unreactive and fixed to light; pupil constriction secondary to hypothalamic or metabolic dysfunction retains reactivity to light.

Continuing observation

It is paramount that the plan of care for head-injured patients continues into the secondary care environment whether this is a general ward or specialist unit. The minimum standard includes: regular recording of the GCS, pupil size and reactivity, respiratory rate, heart rate, blood pressure, temperature and blood oxygen saturation. NICE (2003) have identified that observations should be performed and recorded half-hourly until the GCS is equal to 15. Once a GCS of 15 is achieved, the frequency of observations is identified in Box 8.8.

Scenario 8.2 Skull fracture

Mark Alexander, a 24-year-old male, presents after being hit on the head by a lump of metal, which had fallen from a scaffolding pole. His face, sweater and hands are covered in dried blood and he has a towel wrapped around his head, he appears slightly pale.

His respiratory rate is 14 and regular. His radial pulse is strong and regular and recorded as 54 bpm with a CRT within two seconds. His blood pressure is recorded as 132/74. Mr Alexander complains of having a severe pain to the occipital region of his head and states that it is bleeding profusely. His GCS is recorded as 15/15. His pupils are equal and reactive to light and recorded as 4mm.

He has no relevant medical history.

D *Data* (**scientific facts**): Mr Alexander's presentation is an excellent example of how important the triage process is. An inexperienced staff member may feel that this patient only has a minor injury and with the aid of a few sutures could be discharged. The experienced clinician focuses on the mechanism of injury or risk potential in combination with the presenting clinical condition of the patient.

On presentation, Mr Alexander's observations appear within the normal range. His respiratory rate and rhythm are providing adequate oxygenation; this is confirmed by the lack of cyanosis or a clammy appearance. His pulse rate, although technically bradycardic, is representative of a fit young man and not uncommon, this will, however, need to be monitored as it could be indicative of a cranial haematoma formation. His blood pressure is slightly raised in comparison to the pulse rate and again should be monitored although both blood pressure and pulse are probably completely normal.

The GCS is initially normal with the patient being able to understand and react to verbal stimuli. There are no other obvious signs of injury apart from the head wound, which will need cleaning and exploration as part of the initial assessment.

According to the head injury guidelines (NICE 2003), Mr Alexander does not require a CT scan, he does, however, require a full assessment to identify other risk factors.

E *Emotions* (**intuition**): Mr Alexander's presentation may herald little excitement with him being discharged after his cervical spine has been cleared of injury and the cleaning and closing of a potentially minor head injury which forms the bread and butter work of any emergency department; conversely, on further examination he may be seen to have a hidden skull fracture, therefore his presentation should be taken seriously until high risk factors are negated.

Although he can be admitted to the minor injury area of an emergency department, oxygen and suction should be readily available.

A *Advantages*: Mr Alexander will be fully assessed within one hour, during which time the head wound must be inspected. On inspection there is a large open wound communicating with the skull. Hair should be removed from close proximity to the wound to aid visualization. The skull is palpated to feel for areas of bogginess, pain or areas of inconsistency.

D *Disadvantages* (**differential diagnosis**): a missed skull fracture could have dire consequences for the patient: further damage development, meningitis or osteomyelitis are all possible consequences. In this scenario the skull wound is examined and risk factors identified. If the skull is compromised, the meningeal layers may still be intact providing integral protection. If indicated, a CT scan will direct or rationalize further treatment.

Conclusion

As an emergency care clinician you will encounter patients attending with a head injury on a daily basis. The majority will spend a few hours in the department, be treated, potentially sober up and be safe to discharge. The minority will be assessed and a significant risk identified. These patients will be admitted for regular neurological observation and discharged after senior examination. A very small minority will go on to have varying degrees of brain damage and physical disability due to both their initial accident, and the secondary complications; some will also die as a direct result of either primary or secondary damage.

Good clinical practice, directed in a multi-disciplinary format, can have a significant effect on the patient's prognosis and should not be underestimated.

Patients should only be discharged once all physical symptoms are resolved and suitable supervision at their destination identified. Head injury advice should always be given to patients and their carers before discharge.

9   Respiratory emergencies

Cliff Evans and Emma Tippins

Introduction

This chapter focuses on emergency presentations linked to a change in the individual's ability to breathe. Difficulty in breathing, shortness of breath and dyspnoea are common terms used to describe a patient in respiratory distress. Patients have described the inability to breath (dyspnoea) as a frightening and emotionally upsetting experience (BTS and SIGN 2005). Several acute and chronic pathologies combine to make respiratory-based presentations frequent encounters to all emergency care providers. This chapter will commence with a brief overview of the relevant anatomy and physiology of the respiratory system before progressing onto the assessment of respiratory function. Commonly used airway adjuncts and oxygen delivery devices will be highlighted to provide an evidence base to clinicians' practice. The reader will then be introduced to several clinical scenarios to provide real-life examples of acute respiratory presentations including asthma and pneumonia. National guidance on 'best practice' will be used to provide the reader with a structured approach to patient care delivery.

Dyspnoea

It has been estimated that the cause of around 75 per cent of all patients presenting with dyspnoea can be related to a cardiac or pulmonary cause, the most common of which are listed in Box 9.1.

Box 9.1   Common causes of dyspnoea
• Hypersensitivity airway diseases (asthma) • Chronic obstructive airway disease (bronchitis/emphysema) • Congestive cardiac failure • Infection (chest infection/pneumonia) • Pulmonary embolism • Pneumothorax

Anatomy and physiology

The respiratory system consists of several structures, which combine to produce the act of respiration i.e. cellular oxygenation and the elimination of carbon dioxide (Table 9.1). The act of respiration is a continual process that does not require conscious effort as it is affected by both voluntary and involuntary control. Chapter 2 provided a basic outline of breathing and how the chemoreceptors monitor the circulation and, via a feedback mechanism, inform the higher centres about the need to increase or decrease the rate or depth of respiration in order to maintain homeostasis.

Table 9.1   Form and function of the respiratory system

Form	Structure	Function
Nose	• Composed of cartilage • Lined with a ciliated mucous membrane • The nasal cavity connects to the paranasal sinuses also lined with a mucous membrane	• Sensual organ – smell • Warms, moistens air • Cilia – filter dust and foreign particles including bacteria • Mucus secretion is part of the defensive inflammatory system which prevents particles entering the lungs
Pharynx	• Around 12.5cm in length • Composed of muscular and fibrous tissue • Contains the lymphoid pharyngeal tonsils (adenoids)	• Continues the process of warming, filtering and moistening air • Lymphoid tissue filters and eradicates bacteria
Larynx	• Tube-like structure • Commonly referred to as the voice box • Consisting of cartilage rings • Contains the thyroid cartilage	• Maintains voice production • Continues the process of warming, filtering and moistening inspired air

Table 9.1—*continued*

Form	Structure	Function
Trachea	• Continuation of the larynx • Around 10cm in length • Terminates to divide into the two bronchi • Consists of hyaline cartilage (anteriorly) and involuntary muscle (posteriorly)	• Continues the process of warming, filtering and moistening inspired air • Secretes mucus from goblet cells
Bronchi	• Connection points of trachea to lungs • Consist of hyaline cartilage and involuntary muscle	• Passageway for inspired air into the lungs
Bronchioles	• Composed of muscular fibrous and elastic tissue • Continually narrow until they meet the alveoli	• Passageway for inspired air into the lungs
Alveoli	• Composed of squamous epithelial cells • Entwined with blood capillaries	• Point of gaseous exchange • Carbon dioxide is expelled back through the respiratory system and deoxygenated blood is circulated through the alveoli where it obtains oxygen through the process of diffusion
Lungs	• The two lungs are divided into lobes, the right having superior, middle and inferior lobes, the left having just superior and inferior • Lung tissue is composed of the alveoli, blood vessels, elastic connective tissue	• The lungs facilitate the act of breathing • In combination with the muscles of respiration the lungs inspire and expel air
Pleura	• Serous membrane covering each lung • Composed of an inner visceral layer and an outer parietal layer • These layers are separated by a potential space lubricated with serous fluid	• Prevents friction during the two layers as the lungs expand and contract. • Provides structural points for the lungs

This function could not take place without the assistance of the respiratory muscles. The main muscle of respiration is the diaphragm, a large muscular partition that separates the chest cavity from the abdominal contents. Lying beneath the lungs, the diaphragm resembles a dome shape and stretches across the base of the chest, attaching at various points to bone for stabilization. In combination with the accessory muscles of respiration, air is drawn in by active contraction of the thorax, during inhalation the diaphragm contracts downward and away from the lungs, creating more space in the chest cavity. This lowers the air pressure in the chest cavity relative to the pressure outside the body, subsequently air moves into the lungs. The diaphragm works in combination with the muscles of the neck which attach to the upper part of the sternum and clavicles; the sternocleidomastoid muscle, and the muscles between the ribs; the internal and external intercostal muscles, these increase the diameter of the chest wall, decreasing the pressure in the chest. The intercostal muscles then relax and shrink the chest wall during exhalation.

Airway assessment and management

Without an adequate constant supply of oxygen the patient will soon demonstrate signs of hypoxia. If a patient fails to maintain airway patency, oxygen will not reach the lungs leading to asphyxia. Prevention of hypoxaemia requires a protected, unobstructed flow of air to the lungs with a constant supply of blood and adequate ventilation (Chapter 3). In the patient who is unable to maintain this independently, prompt assessment, with control of the airway and provision of ventilation, is essential.

Airway compromise may be sudden and complete, insidious and partial, and progressive and/or recurrent (American College of Surgeons 2004). It can occur at any level from the nose and mouth down to the bronchi. The site of obstruction varies dependent on the cause; in the unconscious patient the most common cause of airway obstruction is by the posterior displacement of the tongue at the level of the pharynx (RCUK 2006). Vomit, blood, and foreign bodies commonly obstruct airflow at the site of the soft palate and epiglottis resulting in aspiration of particles into the lungs. Obstruction also occurs at the larynx; as a result of inflammation from burns and anaphylaxis, or laryngeal spasm caused by upper airway stimulation or inhalation of foreign bodies. Obstruction below the larynx is also possible, but less common, and can be caused by excessive bronchial secretions, mucosal oedema, bronchospasm, pulmonary oedema, or aspiration of gastric contents.

Airway assessment

Assessment of the patient for signs of airway obstruction is best achieved by the look, listen, feel approach;

- *Look* for chest and abdominal movements
- *Listen* and
- *Feel* for airflow at the mouth and nose.

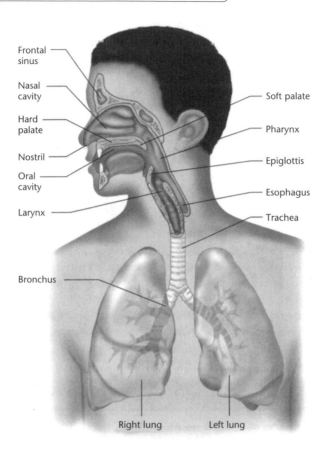

Frontal sinus

Nasal cavity

Hard palate

Nostril

Oral cavity

Larynx

Bronchus

Soft palate

Pharynx

Epiglottis

Esophagus

Trachea

Right lung

Left lung

Source: Shire et al. (2004)

Figure 9.1 Organs of the respiratory system

To effectively assess, put the side of your face, and ear, above the patient's nose and mouth, with your eyes facing the patient's feet; this allows for assessment of all three components in one action.

Signs of airway obstruction can include stridor, wheeze, gurgling, snoring or crowing (Table 9.2).

Many patients present with chronically abnormal and inefficient breathing techniques such as paradoxical chest and abdominal movements, where there is an over-use of the accessory muscles of respiration due to ineffective use of the diaphragm, leaving the neck and shoulder muscles working excessively in opening the lung area to allow oxygen in. This pattern can also be demonstrated in complete airway obstruction resulting in a 'see-saw' or swinging respiratory pattern as the chest wall moves inwards during

Table 9.2 Recognition of airway obstruction

Sign	Cause
Inspiratory stridor	Obstruction at laryngeal level or above
Expiratory wheeze	Obstruction of the lower airways, which can collapse and obstruct during expiration
Gurgling	Presence of liquid or semi-solid foreign material in the upper airways
Snoring	Partial occlusion of the pharynx by the tongue or palate
Crowing or stridor	Laryngeal spasm or obstruction

inspiration, and outwards during expiration. This paradoxical movement is the opposite of the normal respiratory pattern, the result of a high negative intrathoracic pressure being generated against a closed airway.

Airway management

If airway obstruction has been recognized, immediate action must be taken. There are three basic manoeuvres that can be used to relieve upper airway obstruction: head tilt, chin lift and jaw thrust, protecting the cervical spine if necessary (Chapter 5). These simple positional methods are successful in most cases where the cause of the obstruction is loss of muscle tone in the pharynx, however, it is imperative that following any manoeuvre the patient's ability to ventilate is reassessed using the look, listen and feel method described earlier. In cases where a clear airway cannot be achieved, further action is needed. Suction should be used if there is any visible debris in the mouth, suction should only be used in the areas of the oral cavity that can be visualized, pushing a suction catheter down an airway can stimulate a conscious patient's gag reflex, and cause vomiting, exacerbating the problem.

Basic airway adjuncts

Simple airway adjuncts are readily available in all EDs and should be easily accessible as they are helpful, and sometimes essential, in maintaining a patent airway. There are two basic airway adjuncts available to the practitioner: the oropharyngeal and nasopharyngeal airways. These types of airway adjuncts are designed to rectify soft palate obstruction and backward tongue displacement.

The oropharyngeal/Guedel airway is inserted into the mouth behind the tongue. The Guedel airway should be sized prior to insertion; this can be achieved by holding the flange of the airway level with the patient's incisors and the other end of the airway at the angle of the patient's jaw. There are two techniques for insertion, the first is to insert the airway into the oral cavity in the 'upside down' position as far as the junction between the hard and soft palate, and then rotate it through 180 degrees. The other method is to use a tongue blade to depress the tongue and then insert the airway posteriorly. The advantage of the first method is that it minimizes the chance of pushing the tongue backwards and downwards (RCUK 2006). The oropharyngeal airway must not be used in the conscious patient because, again it may induce gagging, vomiting and aspiration. Correct placement is indicated by an improvement in airway patency assessed by using the look, listen, feel approach as before. If an improvement is noted, supplementary oxygen should then be delivered via a facemask with reservoir bag.

The nasopharyngeal airway is utilized in patients who are not deeply unconscious as it is better tolerated than an oropharyngeal airway for reasons described above. The RCUK (2006) recommends sizes 6–7mm as suitable for use in adults, this follows previous techniques, which involved relating the diameter of the little finger to the anatomy of the airway which proved incorrect. Prior to inserting the nasopharyngeal airway, the right nostril should be visualized for patency and absence of nasal polyps, blood or septal deviation, if any of these are present, the other nostril can be checked or another method of securing the airway should be considered. In some designs a safety pin should be inserted into the flanged end prior to insertion to prevent the adjunct disappearing into the airway. A water-soluble lubricant should be used to reduce localized trauma, and then the airway inserted bevel first, vertically along the floor of the nose, twisting gently as this is done. Once the airway is in place and the flange is sitting at the opening of the nostril, reassessment of the airway and breathing should occur with the look, listen, feel approach and supplementary oxygen applied as before. Insertion of the nasopharyngeal airway can cause damage to the mucosal lining of the nasal airway and will result in minor bleeding in 30 per cent of patients (RCUK 2006). Extreme caution should be used when considering the use of the nasopharyngeal airway in patients with obvious, severe facial fractures and suspected basal skull fractures, as passage of the airway through a fracture of the skull base and into the cranial vault is possible, although extremely rare.

In patients demonstrating potential airway compromise, immediate specialist referral is indicated. If at any stage the patency of the airway cannot be maintained the patient will need to be intubated. This definitive procedure should only be undertaken by those qualified in doing so.

Oxygen delivery devices

Box 9.2   Oxygen delivery devices

Oxygen delivery devices are produced in two formats. First, fixed flow and, second, non-fixed flow.

Type of mask:
1 *Fixed flow devices*
• Venturi adaptors

Percentage of oxygen delivered:
• These devices deliver fixed flow oxygen dependent on which adaptor is used, range between 24–60%

2 *Non-fixed flow devices*
• Nebulizing mask
• Ambu bag
• Nasal cannula
• Standard oxygen mask (Hudson)
• Oxygen mask with reservoir bag

Estimated percentage:
• 60% at 6–10 L/min
• 85% at 12–15 L/min
• 24% at 2 L/min (higher rates not recommended)
• 60% at 6–10L/min
• 85% at 10–15L/min

Scenario 9.1   Asthma

James Davies is a 24-year-old Caucasian male who self-presents to the emergency department suffering from a shortness of breath, which he states commenced two hours ago while he was painting his living room. He is unable to complete a full sentence without coughing or stopping briefly to inspire.

His respiratory rate is shallow, rapid and regular at 28 breaths each minute. He has an audible wheeze on expiration and does not appear to be over-using the accessory muscles of respiration. There are no signs of central or peripheral cyanosis. His pulse oximetry reading is 94 per cent on air. His radial pulse is strong, regular and recorded as 129 bpm, CRT is within two seconds. The initial blood pressure is recorded as 132/87.

Mr Davies appears anxious, sweaty and clammy. He is orientated to time and place, with an AVPU score of A.

Relevant medical history includes eczema and asthma for which he takes a Salbutamol inhaler as required.

D *Data* (scientific facts): Mr Davies presents with several early warning signs of respiratory compromise that may lead to respiratory failure. His respiratory rate of 28, in conjunction with a pulse rate above 110, demonstrates compensatory shock. The British Thoracic Society (BTS) clarification of the severity of asthma can be found in Figure 9.2. This assessment and management

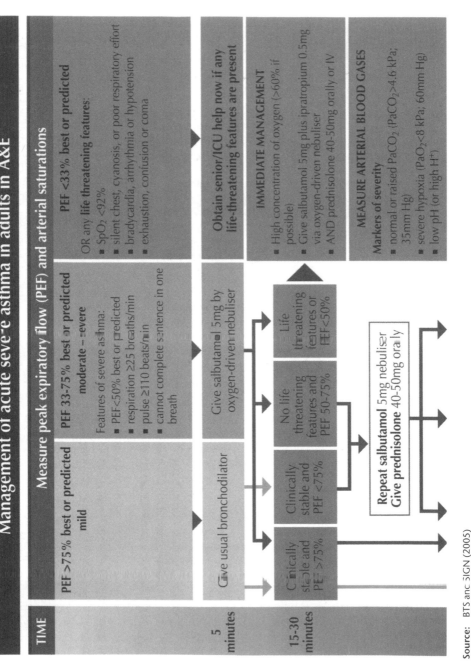

Management of acute severe asthma in adults in A&E

Measure peak expiratory flow (PEF) and arterial saturations

TIME				
	PEF >75% best or predicted mild	**PEF 33-75% best or predicted** moderate – severe Features of severe asthma: ■ PEF <50% best or predicted ■ respiration ≥25 breaths/min ■ pulse ≥110 beats/min ■ cannot complete sentence in one breath	**PEF <33% best or predicted** OR any life threatening features: ■ SpO₂ <92% ■ silent chest, cyanosis, or poor respiratory effort ■ bradycardia, arrhythmia or hypotension ■ exhaustion, confusion or coma	
5 minutes	Give usual bronchodilator	Give salbutamol 5mg by oxygen-driven nebuliser	**Obtain senior/ICU help now if any life-threatening features are present**	
15-30 minutes			**IMMEDIATE MANAGEMENT** ■ High concentration of oxygen (>60% if possible) ■ Give salbutamol 5mg plus ipratropium 0.5mg via oxygen-driven nebuliser ■ AND prednisolone 40-50mg orally or IV	

Clinically stable and PEF >75%

Clinically stable and PEF <75%

No life threatening features and PEF 50-75%

Life threatening features or PEF <50%

Repeat salbutamol 5mg nebuliser
Give prednisolone 40-50mg orally

MEASURE ARTERIAL BLOOD GASES
Markers of severity
■ normal or raised PaCO₂ (PaCO₂>4.6 kPa; 35mm Hg)
■ severe hypoxia (PaO₂<8 kPa; 60mm Hg)
■ low pH (or high H⁺)

Source: BTS and SIGN (2005)

Figure 9.2   Management of acute severe asthma in A&E

60 minutes

120 minutes

| Patient recovering and PEF >75% | No signs of severe asthma and PEF 50-75% | Signs of severe asthma or PEF <50% |

Signs of severe asthma or PEF <50%:
- Give/repeat salbutamol 5mg with ipratropium 0.5mg by oxygen-driven nebuliser after 15 mins
- Consider continuous salbutamol nebuliser 5-10mg/hr
- Consider IV magnesium sulphate 1.2-2g over 20 minutes
- Correct fluid/electrolytes, especially K^+ disturbances
- Chest x-ray

ADMIT
Patient should be accompanied by a nurse or doctor at all times

Observe
monitor SpO_2, heart rate and respiratory rate

Signs of severe asthma or PEF <50%

Patient stable and PEF >50%

POTENTIAL DISCHARGE
- In all patients who received nebulised β_2 agonists prior to presentation, consider an extended observation period prior to discharge
- If PEF <50% on presentation, prescribe prednisolone 40-50mg/day for 5 days
- In all patients, ensure treatment supply of inhaled steroid and β_2 agonist and check inhaler technique
- Arrange GP follow up for 2 days post presentation
- Fax discharge letter to GP
- Refer to asthma liaison nurse/chest clinic

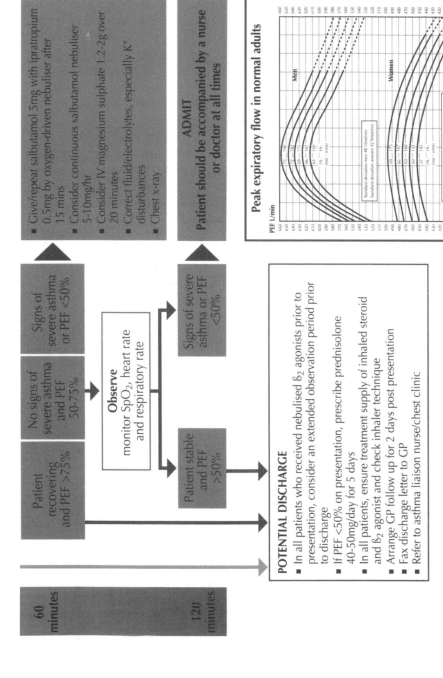

Peak expiratory flow in normal adults

Thorax 2003; **58** (Suppl I): i1-i92

algorithm focuses on the use of quantifiable data to justify treatment. In this case the three indicators of severe compromise are the respiratory and pulse rates and the low oxygen saturation level. Clinically this is evident by his sweaty and clammy appearance.

Mr Davies has an atopic history, which means he has a predisposition to various hypersensitivity reactions such as asthma, eczema and rhinitis. Clinicians should proceed with caution when treating these patients with medications, particularly with intravenous antibiotics, due to the high correlation between atopic individuals and anaphylactic reactions to common antibiotics, namely penicillin and cephalosporins.

E *Emotions* (**intuition**): from the primary data gathered Mr Davies appears to be experiencing an asthma attack related to his exposure to antigens from the paint fumes which he inhaled. Mr Davies should be placed in an area of the emergency department with the facilities to intubate if necessary as his presentation is severe, and if initial treatment fails, he may deteriorate into respiratory failure and ultimately respiratory arrest.

A *Advantages*: the application of high flow supplementary oxygen is essential; this should be combined with nursing the patient in a sitting position, allowing full lung expansion. Therapy should be continually monitored via regular assessment of respiratory effort and rate, which should be documentation in combination with pulse oximetry. Mr Davies will require a peak expiratory flow (PEF) recording, which will further substantiate his level of respiratory compromise and guide the effectiveness of treatments. A PEF meter records the maximum flow of air that can be expelled in one single expiration, it provides a convenient indicator of the amount of bronchial constriction, although readings can be affected by a poor user technique, Box 9.3 describes

---

Box 9.3 Recording peak expiratory flow rates

Many patients with a history of asthma will undertake regular peak flow recordings at home and will know their expected score; note this but be aware of their technique.

There are several meters on the market and patients are usually advised to keep their meter and to bring it with them if they attend hospital to reduce cross-infection rates. A disposable tube should be placed on the mouthpiece, the meter reset to zero and held by the patient horizontally. The patient should be directed to take a deep breath in before placing the meter in their mouth. Their lips should be applied to the mouthpiece and the air expelled in one hard, fast breath. If the breath is continual and not short and sharp, it may induce coughing. This test should be repeated three times and the highest score recorded. If possible, record their PEFR pre and post any nebulized interventions, as this will provide quantifiable data to the effectiveness of treatments.

how to take a PEF reading. Mr Davis's lungs will need auscultation by an appropriately trained individual to ascertain if infection is present or whether a chest X-ray is necessary.

Many emergency departments and ambulance services have local protocols in relation to acute asthma presentations, and these are generally related to the administration of a beta2 agonist, such as Salbutamol, which will relax the smooth muscle of the bronchioles and correct some of the airway narrowing or spasm. In combination with supplementary oxygen, this therapy may completely curtail the patient's symptoms.

D *Disadvantages* (**differential diagnosis**): a spontaneous pneumothorax, depending on the level of lung compromise, can present in a similar way to an acute asthma attack. Chest auscultation may identify the possibility of more insidious pathologies or coexisting disease. It is not common practice to order routine chest X-rays in these patients, due to both unnecessary exposure to a lifetime of radiation and the cost and resource impact. When a patient presents with wheezing, a systemic allergic reaction should be negated, as the presenting symptoms may be similar, look for laryngeal oedema, urticaria, and hypotension (Chapter 2).

Asthma

Definition and prevalence

Asthma can be defined as a chronic condition with acute exacerbations resulting in a hypersensitivity reaction. Asthma is a multi-dimensional phenomenon in which the culmination of the hypersecretion of mucus, constriction of smooth muscle within the bronchioles and localized inflammation result in the affected individual's ability to breathe becoming compromised. The Global Initiative for Asthma (GINA 2004) estimate that 300 million people, of all ages and races, experience asthma, and the annual incidence is increasing in all age groups. GINA estimate that asthma accounts for one in 250 deaths worldwide, many of which are preventable, suboptimal long-term medical care and delay in seeking help are the main contributing factors.

Industrialized countries top the list of worldwide prevalence with Scotland currently demonstrating a prevalence rate of 18 per cent, England 15 per cent and the United States of America 11 per cent (GINA 2004). The UK demonstrates the worst prevalence rate in Europe in comparison to Sweden's 6 per cent and Denmark's 3 per cent, however, the UK has a mortality rate of around 3 per cent which is extremely low in comparison to China's 36 per cent or Denmark's 9 per cent. There are many theories related to the causes of asthma (Currie et al. 2005) although no one factor appears solely responsible.

Assessment

The indicative signs or symptoms of asthma are an expiratory wheeze, sometimes combined with wheezing on inspiration, shortness of breath, chest tightness and coughing. These symptoms are variable, intermittent, worse at night and can be provoked by certain triggers, or allergens, in the form of dust mites or pollen, chemical allergens such as paint fumes, or exercise and cold weather. In addition psychological components have been extensively implicated in provoking an acute asthma attack (BTS and SIGN 2005).

When a patient presents in an alert and orientated condition, the assessment can begin by observing the patient's respiratory rate, depth and the amount of effort the patient is using to achieve effective respiration. The term 'effort' centres on the use of the shoulder girdle to assist breathing, patients frequently present resting forward, with their arms outstretched which braces the shoulder girdle allowing for the use of the accessory muscles of respiration, the sternocleidomastoid and trapezius muscles being the most evident. The ability of the patient to talk is a prime discriminator of serious illness; if the patient is able to talk in full sentences, it is highly unlikely that a serious airway compromise is present.

Patients with an established history of asthma may know their usual best PEF and this will provide a baseline for evaluation of their condition. Current PEF recordings will be expressed as a percentage of the patient's previous best. If this information is unavailable, the PEF should be documented as a percentage of their predicted rate; this can be achieved by using the graph predictor in Figure 9.2. The continual monitoring of the patient's respiratory rate and oxygen saturation by pulse oximetry will determine the effectiveness of the supplementary oxygen therapy, as arterial blood gas is indicated if the SpO_2 falls below 92 per cent.

Physiological findings comprise the majority of the initial assessment, although there are other influencing factors. The BTS guidelines (2005) state that in the assessment of asthma the assessor should note if the patient presents with one or more psychosocial factors such as psychiatric illness (depression), or drug and alcohol use, as these patients have a significantly increased mortality rate (BTS and SIGN 2005).

Treatment options

There is no universal approach to the prevention and management of asthma, with both the United Kingdom and United States of America classifying the severity of asthma in different ways (Cates 2001). The UK philosophy focuses on prevention with the stepwise approach (BTS and SIGN 2005). This approach centres on increasing the use of medications depending on the frequency and severity of symptoms and exacerbations, beginning with the use of inhaled short-acting Beta2 agonists, as required, for mild inter-mittent episodes, through to the daily use of oral and inhaled steroids. Recent pharmalogical advances have led to the development of preventative medications, which aim to prevent, or antagonize a major component, or instigator of asthma, these are the leukotriene antagonists.

The treatment of acute exacerbations such as in the case of Mr Davies follows the BTS and SIGN guidelines (2005) (Figure 9.2). The clinical symp-toms associated with the presentation of Mr Davies indicate a moderate–severe presentation. These presentations frequently resolve with the administration of high-flow oxygen and nebulized Beta2 agonists, which should be delivered within five minutes of the patient assessment. If the symptoms resolve and the PEF returns to above 75 per cent of the patient's predicted score, the patient can be discharged. If the patient's clinical condition slightly improves but the PEF remains under 75 per cent of the expected range, a repeat Beta2 agonist should be nebulized and the patient commenced on oral steroid therapy. By strictly adhering to the guidelines this reassessment will take place within 30 mins and can be re-evaluated within the hour. If at any point the patient's clinical condition deteriorates, more intensive therapy should begin. This section of the algorithm includes the administration of ipratropium, an anti-cholinergic bronchodilator, recording and measuring arterial blood gases, and possible administration of magnesium and intubation if medication does not improve the patient's condition (Figure 9.2).

This structured assessment and management tool will have a profound positive effect in clinical practice as novice practitioners have a solid frame-work from which to practise. All clinicians, regardless of discipline, should familiarize themselves with the guidelines as quick and effective action can prevent patient deterioration.

Chronic obstructive pulmonary disease (COPD)

Scenario 9.2 COPD

Freda Swartz is a 78-year-old female who is brought into the emergency depart-ment at 04.45 experiencing a sudden severe episode of shortness of breath. She is unable to complete a sentence although she appears lucid.

Her respiratory rate is shallow, rapid and regular at 38 breaths each minute.

She appears to be over-using the accessory muscle of respiration, her neck veins are protruding and she adopts the tripod position (sitting, leaning forward with arms on thighs), and there is evidence of peripheral cyanosis. Her radial pulse is strong, irregular and recorded as 92 bpm, CRT is within two seconds. The initial blood pressure is recorded as 148/92. Mrs Swartz appears pale, sweaty and clammy. She is orientated to time and place, with an AVPU score of A.

Past medical history includes atrial fibrillation for which she takes Digoxin. Mrs Swartz is a chronic smoker of around 20 cigarettes a day and has been an inpatient on several occasions with similar presentations related to what she describes as a chronic breathing problem. She is producing purulent sputum, when questioned, she states she commonly produces thick yellow or green phlegm particularly in the mornings.

D *Data* (scientific facts): primary data indicate a potentially life-threatening presentation. This is demonstrated by her inability to complete a sentence, an ominous sign of impending respiratory failure. The dramatic rise in the patient's respiratory rate confirms the initial clinical findings.

Her pulse and blood pressure are raised, which in conjunction with the normal CRT indicates an adequate circulation. A respiratory cause is therefore highly likely.

Her past medical history includes a possible compromise of her cardiovascular system, therefore a pre-existing or acute cardiac-related episode would need to be negated.

E *Emotions* (intuition): established heart disease and a patient demonstrating obvious hypoxia should trigger warning signs to the experienced clinician, leading to the immediate request for senior assistance and transfer of the patient into the resuscitation room. The patient also has a chronic history of smoking, which may indicate more serious internal compromise of both the cardiovascular and respiratory systems.

A *Advantages*: as with all serious presentations, high-flow oxygen should be administered, regardless of whether the patient may have a history of chronic obstructive pulmonary disease (COPD). The application of high-flow supplementary oxygen is essential until proven otherwise (RCUK 2006) (Box 9.5). The patient should be assisted to sit upright to reduce the work of breathing, this may involve the use of several pillows or rolled blankets. The effectiveness of treatments should be closely monitored and evaluated; this will involve continually monitoring the patient's oxygen saturation level via a pulse oximeter, and regular respiratory rate assessment and documentation.

In this scenario when the lungs are auscultated, there is evidence of consolidation, crackles and wheezing; this indicates a mixed collection of pathologies, which is often the case in older patients. A chest X-ray should be requested to assist decision-making with regards to future management of Mrs Swartz.

An intravenous cannula will need to be sited and bloods obtained; these should include a blood sugar as patients with a chronic history of presentations for respiratory compromise may develop diabetes due to the repeated use of steroids.

An arterial blood gas may be necessary to identify the origin of the illness and its effect on the body. The patient will need to be connected to cardiac monitoring and a 12-lead ECG recorded. Her temperature will also need to be recorded and monitored.

D *Disadvantages* (**differential diagnosis**): patients presenting with severe respiratory compromise in the early hours of the morning are a common event in acute services. When a patient has a known cardiac history the obvious cause is that they have slipped down into a flatter sleeping position during the night, causing pulmonary oedema; this inability to breathe while lying flat is termed orthopnoea. Orthopnoea is most commonly associated with heart failure, but is also seen in asthma and chronic bronchotic conditions. The slow insidious developments of a chest infection and eventually pneumonia, or the exacerbation of COPD, are examples of potential relevant disease processes. Distended neck veins may indicate a problem with blood flow into the heart, which could be due to heart failure or a tension pneumothorax, both of which will need negating.

The immediate management, regardless of the aetiology, is to maintain oxygenation and an adequate circulation. In other words, if in doubt of a diagnosis, return to the underlying principles of the ABCDE assessment. Both COPD and heart failure share many of the same physical signs; therefore an initial diagnosis may be compromised leading to a delay in appropriate treatment. Kleinschmidt (2005) suggests a crude bedside test for distinguishing COPD from heart failure, which centres on recording a PEF. If the patient scores below 200ml, they are probably having an exacerbation of COPD, PEF above 200, however, may indicate an exacerbation of heart failure.

A sputum sample should be sent to microbiology to ascertain the infective agent enabling appropriate antibiotics to be prescribed. All patients presenting with sporadic bouts of coughing and purulent sputum production should be risk-assessed for tuberculosis, as this infection could be spread to other users of the emergency department or to healthcare professionals.

COPD: definition and prevalence

COPD can be defined as a chronic and debilitating disease continuum in which localized irritation of the bronchioles and lungs results in increasing airflow obstruction. COPD encompasses several lung conditions with varying causes, although smoking is by far the most significant factor in its development (NICE 2004).

It is estimated that 900,000 individuals are diagnosed with COPD in the UK alone and this disease process accounts for around 30,000 deaths each year (NICE 2004).

In the United States of America there are an estimated 32 million affected individuals, with COPD being the fourth leading cause of death (Kleinschmidt 2003). Worldwide COPD is the sixth leading cause of death.

Pathophysiology

COPD is a combination of three separate disease processes that culminate to complete the clinical and pathophysiological picture of lung disease (the two major components are identified in Box 9.4). These disease processes are chronic bronchitis, emphysema, and to a lesser extent, chronic asthma. Each individual experiencing COPD has a unique mixture of these three instigators.

Symptoms are insidious and usually begin to appear later in life. The early warning signs or symptoms are the excessive production of phlegm and a chronic cough generally lasting in excess of three months. The diagnosis of COPD should be considered in all patients over 35 who have a chronic history of smoking, and who present with external breathlessness, a chronic cough and regular sputum production (NICE 2004). The formal diagnosis of COPD is confirmed by spirometry.

Due to the underlying disease process patients with COPD are susceptible to many pathologies that can result in a rapid deterioration of their already chronically compromised lung function. The NICE have produced specific guidelines for the treatment and management of this group of individuals (NICE 2004) (Figure 9.3).

Treatment options

The initial management of exacerbations of COPD centre on the use of nebulized bronchodilators, supplementary oxygen and antibiotics if the patient is producing purulent sputum. When tachypnoea is a prominent feature, steroids should be added to the therapy, these are continued for one to two weeks and tailed off to prevent an acute adrenal insufficiency crisis.

Maintenance of the patient's oxygen saturation above 90 per cent is essential, this will be achieved by supplementing oxygen and dilating the bronchioles, in addition, steroids will begin to reduce the inflammation and anti-cholinergic bronchodilators will reduce mucus secretion. The need for non-invasive therapy or intubation should be stratified and the opinion of a senior anaesthetist should be sought, in the prevailing period a respiratory stimulant could be commenced, particularly if the patient's level of consciousness begins to decrease.

Non-invasive ventilation

Non-invasive ventilation is a key component to treating severe presentations of COPD. The underpinning rationale to non-invasive ventilation is to correct

---

Box 9.4 The main instigators of COPD

Chronic bronchitis:
Chronic bronchial inflammation (bronchitis) leads to continuous stimulation of the immune system resulting in an excessive production of mucus and hyperplasia of mucus-producing glands resulting in the obstructive component of chronic bronchitis.

The internal response is to increase the cardiac output and decrease ventilation, thereby producing a ventilation perfusion mismatch leading to hypoxaemia hypercapnia and a mixture of respiratory and metabolic acidosis. Heart failure is a common pre-existing factor as the chronic respiratory failure causes pulmonary hypertension, and right heart enlargement (cor-pulmonale). These patients have traditionally been described as 'blue bloaters' due to the clinical picture that these disease processes culminate in.

Emphysema:
Emphysema is defined as a destruction of the distal airways. The alveoli and capillary beds that entwine them are gradually destroyed leading to the inability to oxygenate blood.

The internal environment compensates by increasing ventilation and lowering the cardiac output, resulting in hypoxia. Due to the excessive respiratory function individuals experience chronic weight loss and muscle wasting. Traditionally described as 'pink puffers'.

Clinical presentation

Chronic bronchitis:
- Patients may be obese
- Frequent cough and expectoration are typical
- Use of accessory muscles of respiration is common
- The breath sounds are often normal but upon auscultation there may be inspiratory and expiratory crackles, rhonchi (coarse gurgling) and wheezes
- Patients may have signs of right heart failure (i.e., cor pulmonale), such as oedema and cyanosis
- Similar overall appearance to heart failure.

Emphysema:
- Patients may be very thin with a barrel-shaped chest (hyper-inflated)
- They typically have little or no cough or expectoration
- Breathing may be assisted by pursed lips and use of accessory respiratory muscles; they may adopt the tripod sitting position
- The chest may be hyper-resonant, and wheezing may be heard
- Overall appearance is more like classic COPD exacerbation

---

hypoventilation and reduce the workload of the accessory respiratory muscles; this is achieved by forcing open distal areas of lung space. The use of continuous positive airway pressure (CPAP) has been shown to be an effective frontline treatment and all emergency department personnel should be familiar with its application (Vanpee et al. 2002). The major drawback of

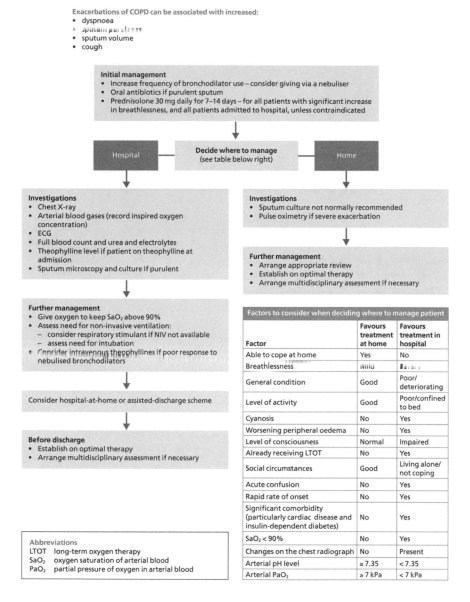

Source: NICE (2004)

Figure 9.3 Managing exacerbations of COPD

this therapy is that many patients find it hard to tolerate, although newer machines incorporate a pressure sensor to enable the machine to alter the CPAP pressure on a breath-by-breath basis, thereby making it more tolerable.

If this therapy fails to improve the patient's condition within 30 minutes, the patient may need intubation (Poponick et al. 1999). Another current therapy is the use of heliox, a mixture of helium and oxygen. Heliox has been seen to reduce the amount of work the patient needs to make in expiring, thereby reducing the overall respiratory effort (Johnson et al. 2002).

Box 9.5   Oxygen therapy: myths and reality

- Adequate oxygen should be given to relieve all cases of hypoxia.
- In COPD aim to maintain SpO_2 > 90–93 per cent
- It is widely believed that supplementing too much oxygen can cause significant respiratory depression: multiple studies dispute this as administrating high-flow oxygen causes PO_2 and PCO_2 to rise, but not in proportion to the very minor changes in respiratory drive (Kleinschmidt 2005).
- Increased circulating PCO_2 can occasionally precipitate a decrease in the patient's level of consciousness; a subsequent reduction in supplementary oxygen only leads to profound hypoxia.
- Patients exhibiting clinical deterioration should either receive a trial of non-invasive ventilation or be intubated.

Pneumonia

Scenario 9.3   Pneumonia

Mrs Fairfield, an 82-year-old Caucasian female, presents with a five-day history of increasing shortness of breath and lethargy. She is accompanied by her two daughters who are very upset about the care she has received so far from her general practitioner (GP) who refused to visit her at home. She had previously been seen by her GP who had prescribed her amoxycillin for a chest infection.

Mrs Fairfield looks unwell, although she is able to complete a sentence. Her respiratory rate is 23, shallow and regular. The distal aspects of her fingers are cyanosed although there is no evidence of central cyanosis. Her pulse is strong, regular and recorded as 129bpm, with a CRT of four seconds. The initial blood pressure is recorded as 84/49.

Mrs Fairfield appears pale, is orientated to time and place, with an AVPU score of A. Although she feels hot, her temperature is 36 degrees centigrade.

Mrs Fairfield's past medical history includes hypertension for which she takes atenolol, amlodapine and simvastatin.

D *Data* (scientific facts): primary data indicate a serious presentation. This is demonstrated by the compensatory increase in respiratory rate, the reduced capillary refill time, tachycardia and hypotension, which are a cause for concern and may indicate decompensated shock, the most probable cause being pneumonia secondary to a prolonged chest infection.

E *Emotions* (intuition): experienced clinicians are able to add several independent variables together to construct a working diagnosis. The patient's history of increasing shortness of breath and lethargy can indicate ominous signs of impending respiratory failure, thus the patient will therefore be nursed within a high dependency area. Clinical signs reinforce the clinician's intuition that a seriously unwell individual confronts them. Experienced clinicians will also recognize that elderly patients are less likely than younger individuals to demonstrate a temperature in response to severe infection (BTS and SIGN 2005).

A *Advantages*: the patient should be commenced on high flow supplementary oxygen, and an oxygen saturation probe used to monitor its effectiveness, along with regular recording of the respiratory rate, pulse and blood pressure, the early intervention of a physiotherapist may assist in treating lung consolidation and enable the patient to breathe more easily. His or her lungs will need auscultation by an appropriately trained individual to ascertain if infection is present and a chest X-ray will aid the diagnosis of community-acquired pneumonia (CAP) (Figure 9.4).

Other sources of infection should be identified, such as a urinary tract infection.

Intravenous access needs to be gained and blood should be requested in line with the BTS guidelines on the treatment of CAP, these include:

- Full blood count
- Urea and electrolytes
- Liver function test
- C reactive protein

Blood should also be taken for micro-culture and sensitivity before broad spectrum antibiotics are given.

A fluid challenge may aid the blood pressure, although fluid resuscitation generally fails if the patient is septic (Chapter 2). A urinary catheter will need to be inserted and strict measurement of fluid balance instigated.

Due to the history surrounding the presentation, family members may have hesitancy and distrust about the healthcare system due to the treatment he or she has received so far. This should be addressed at an early stage. The family, and potentially the patient, will need reassurance that they have come to the right place and will receive a high standard of quality treatment. The main point should be to focus on the positive aspects of the current treatment plan and not on the negative of their previous encounters.

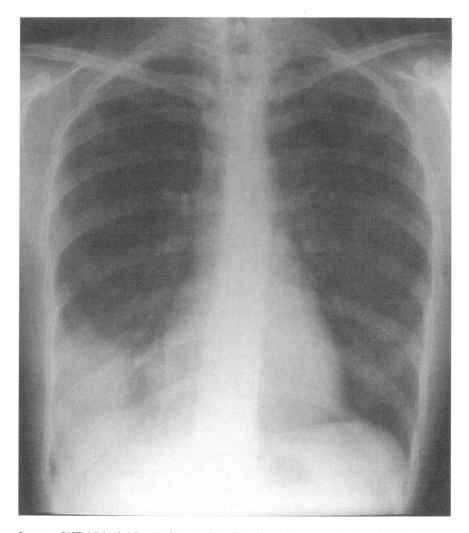

Source: CAPT Michael John Hughey at: http://www.brooksidepress.org/Products/OBGYN_101/My Documents4/Xray/Chest/Pneumonia.htm

Figure 9.4 Right lower lobe pneumonia

D *Disadvantages* (differential diagnosis): many respiratory-based conditions present with similar clinical signs. Exacerbations of COPD, asthma and pulmonary oedema are classic examples; pulmonary embolism, lung cancer and inhaled foreign bodies are other possibilities. The patient's presenting history may reveal subtle clues to the current instigator. Tests will need to be undertaken to pinpoint the current diagnosis and management plan, this is a multi-disciplinary task, with negation of the most serious pathologies the priority.

Pneumonia: definition and prevalence

Pneumonia can be defined as an acute inflammation of the lower respiratory tract most commonly due to viral and bacterial infection. Areas or lobes of the lungs become consolidated resulting in an impairment of gas exchange. The British Thoracic Society guidelines on the management of pneumonia include evidence of radiographic shadowing (BTS 2004).

Classification of pneumonia

Pneumonia is classified into two distinct subgroups; the reason for this is that the two groups, despite having many common features, are treated very differently.

Community-acquired pneumonia
Pneumonia that is contracted outside of the hospital setting often follows a viral respiratory infection; it affects nearly four million adults each year. Community-acquired pneumonia is caused by a small range of bacteria, namely Streptococcus Pneumonie (BTS 2004). Patients within the community are treated empirically, i.e., microbial investigations are not routinely requested and sputum should only be examined if the patient fails to respond to oral antibiotics.

Hospital-acquired pneumonia
Pneumonia that is contracted within the hospital is called nosocomial pneumonia. Hospitalized patients are particularly vulnerable to pneumonia, a complication of bed rest and a leading secondary infection. The main pathogens responsible for disease within the hospital environment are frequently resistant to standard antibiotics. They also prove to be increasingly virulent and associated morbidity and mortality is high. Hospital-acquired pneumonia is the leading cause of death in hospitalized patients. These infections require specific antibiotics depending on the bacteria present; therefore pathogen identification is essential.

The annual incidence of community-acquired pneumonia is 6–34/1000 adults in the United Kingdom (BTS 2004). There is a direct correlation between age and prevalence, with the over-75 age range having a prevalence of 34/1000.

The mortality rate is estimated at around 10 per cent and is the fifth leading cause of death in the UK with elderly patients experiencing the most serious effects (BTS 2004).

Pneumonia is the sixth leading cause of death in the United States and the leading cause of death from an infection; pneumonia is also the leading hospital-acquired infection and cause of death (Pellerano 2005). National guidelines are designed to treat patients within the community where the mortality rates and cost remain lower at around £100 per presentation, within the hospital setting the average cost for treating a patient escalates to between £2000 and £5000, one prime variable affecting these figures may be the severity of the patient's physical condition.

The BTS guidelines identify a 5-point scoring system based on individual clinical features and these are summarized in Box 9.6; the reader is also referred to the guidelines for in-depth reading (BTS 2004).

Box 9.6   The CRB-65 scoring system

Score 1 point for each feature present:

- Confusion
- Urea > 7 mmol/l
- Respiratory rate > 30/min
- Blood pressure Systolic (< 90mmHg) Diastolic (< 60mmHg)
- Age > 65 years

A CURB-65 score of 0 is associated with a mortality rate of 1.2%. This figure rises to 18.2% for a score of 4 (BTS 2004).

- 0–1   Assess suitability for home treatment
- 2   Consider hospital treatment
- 3   Or more, manage as severe pneumonia
- 4–5   Assess need for ITU admission

Pathophysiology

A viral infection can lead to the individual's immune system becoming compromised and creates an ideal opportunity for bacterial proliferation and the subsequent development of pneumonia. The alveoli become inflamed and saturated with fluid. Pneumonia can result from a variety of causes, including infectious agents such as bacteria, viruses, fungi and parasites. In addition, pneumonia may also occur from chemical or physical injury to the lungs. This can include aspirational pneumonia, a common complication of a stroke or compromise to the patency of the protective mechanisms of the airway: altered levels of consciousness, neuromuscular disease or seizures. Inhalation of infectious particles is probably the most important pathogenetic mechanism in the development of community-acquired pneumonia, various pathogens can colonize the lungs and cause disease, for example, tuberculosis.

The clinical signs and features associated with acute pneumonia are insidious and develop over days to weeks.

In hospital-acquired pneumonia, invasive tubes or investigations compromise the anatomical defences (Table 9.1) and result in bacteria bypassing the defence network and directly compromising the tracheobronchial tree via colonization, leading to a massive inflammatory reaction and an increase in mucus production. This escalating reaction results in bacteria entering the bloodstream, causing involvement of the systemic circulation and the affected individual will demonstrate septicaemia. Hospital-acquired pneumonia is therefore far more virulent and destructive.

Treatment

Treatment focuses on administering appropriate antibiotics to terminate the colonization of bacteria, sustaining optimum oxygenation through simultaneously supplementing oxygen and maintaining the mean arterial pressure above 60–5mmHg. Providing humidified oxygen early into the treatment plan will reduce the incidence of damage to the airways and mucous membranes associated with high-flow oxygen administration. The early intervention of specialist care, i.e., ITU and physiotherapy to assist the movement of lung consolidation, will benefit the prognosis. Keeping the patient well hydrated and nourished has also been shown to benefit patient outcomes.

Conclusion

The benefits of applying theory to clinical practice

The ability of frontline clinicians to correctly assess for life-threatening signs of actual, or impending, respiratory compromise is essential. This knowledge and practical skill base is achieved through understanding both the relevant anatomy and pathophysiology of common clinical presentations.

A problem-solving approach is crucial when assessing and implementing treatment for patients experiencing dyspnoea. Once an intervention has taken place, reassessment and evaluation are necessary. Evaluation is easily achieved through regular monitoring of the patient's level of consciousness, respiratory rate and effort of breathing, in addition to the use of pulse oximetry or arterial blood gases depending on the presenting severity.

Familiarizing yourself with the many instruments available to assist the passage of oxygen into the lungs can prove invaluable when confronted with potential and actual airway compromise.

10 Medical emergencies

Cliff Evans

Introduction

Acute presentations related to an underpinning medical problem constitute a large proportion of a modern emergency department's workload. There are countless acute and chronic medical pathologies that could lead to a patient's presentation. This chapter will, therefore, discuss the most serious, or frequent presentations, and those that early expert intervention can have a positive beneficial impression upon. These include cerebral vascular accident (CVA) or stroke, sickle cell disease, upper gastrointestinal (GI) bleeds, pulmonary embolism (PE) and diabetic emergencies.

The use of scenarios and the application of the critical thinking framework will again highlight prominent areas for the clinician to gain insight into. Many of the pathologies are only superficially discussed and, therefore, further in-depth reading is suggested. Recommended reading can be found in the key references section.

Cerebral vascular accident (CVA)

Scenario 10.1   Cerebral vascular accident

Mrs Ambrose, a 64-year-old Afro-Caribbean female, attends the ED following a collapse at home in the kitchen. She had been cooking when she experienced a sudden sharp pain in her head, which she describes as a thunderous noise. The pain has now been replaced by a sensation of numbness.

Her respiratory rate is 21 and regular. There are no signs of central or peripheral cyanosis. Her radial pulse is strong, regular and recorded as 79 bpm, CRT is within two seconds. The initial blood pressure is recorded as 210/117. The patient appears anxious, and although slightly apprehensive, she is lucid. She appears slightly pale, although not sweaty and clammy. She obeys commands and is orientated to time and place, with an AVPU score of A. Her pupils are size 4, equal and reactive to light. She feels warm to touch at both a central and peripheral level.

Relevant medical history includes hypertension for which she takes atenolol, aspirin and garlic.

D *Data* (scientific facts): from the primary data gathered, the patient does not appear to be displaying signs of physiological shock, this is initially identified by the lack of actual, or potential airway compromise, and the respiratory rate is slightly increased, although no evidence of peripheral or central cyanosis is evident. The radial pulse is strong indicating an adequate circulation, confirmed by a distal capillary refill time within two seconds. An oxygen saturation probe and cardiac monitoring should be employed in conjunction with a 12-lead ECG. The patient exhibits severe hypertension despite taking anti-hypertensive medication, making this presentation potentially life-threatening. Despite the warning signs of a CVA, the patient's initial neurological assessment reveals an A, using the AVPU score.

E *Emotions* (intuition): established hypertension places the patient at increased risk of coronary heart disease, stroke and aneurysm development. As stated, this patient has presented with severe hypertension, which, in combination with the sudden sharp non-traumatic head pain the patient felt, could indicate the sinister features associated with a subarachnoid haemorrhage. In this context the hypertension noted could indicate the onset of an increasing intracranial pressure (ICP) secondary to a bleed. The other two cardinal signs of an increased ICP are bradycardia and bradypnoea, when combined; these three signs are referred to as Cushing's triad (Chapter 8). The other classic sign of an internal insult to the brain is a decrease in the individual's level of consciousness (for in-depth details, refer to Chapter 8).

The experienced assessor will sense the need for urgent action due to the presenting patient history. This would lead the clinician to place the patient in a high dependency area of the ED, thereby expediting the patient's care and negating serious illness. This will also allow close monitoring and observation where any deterioration in the patient's clinical condition can be identified.

A *Advantages*: obtaining a thorough history of the circumstances surrounding the presentation, or mechanism of injury, is paramount. This is of particular importance when it involves a patient with a history of high risk factors for serious illness, as the background events may provide subtle clues to the instigating pathology. As with all potentially serious presentations the clinician should commence high-flow oxygen and pulse oximetry. The early insertion of a cannula while the patient is stable is essential, as once the patient begins to deteriorate, the peripheral circulation may be compromised, resulting in an inability to gain intravenous access.

D *Disadvantages* (**differential diagnosis**): when faced with a patient presenting in a stable condition, but with high risk factors for serious illness and a sinister presenting history, the practitioner must take the situation extremely seriously and proceed with caution when making a working diagnosis.

Hypertension

Patients presenting with hypertension fall into two classes: first, individuals who present with various injuries and illness, and as part of the assessment process are identified as having either undiagnosed hypertension or a chronic history of hypertension; second, those presenting with varying states of illness as a direct result of either diagnosed or undiagnosed hypertension. In England, around 34 per cent of men and 30 per cent of females have established hypertension, and it is estimated that, despite treatment, around 60 per cent remain hypertensive (BHF 2006). Hypertension and hyperlipidaemia are significant risk factors for the development of both CVD and CVA (BHF 2006).

CVA/Stroke

Stroke is a medical emergency: a confirmed diagnosis can instigate appropriate treatment similarly to AMI, where time is of the essence. The Stroke Association have championed the 'FAST' acronym of assessment, which is outlined in Box 10.1.

Box 10.1 The FAST acronym

Facial weakness – can the person smile? Has their mouth or eye drooped?
Arm weakness – can the person raise both arms?
Speech problems – can the person speak clearly and understand what you say?
Test all three symptoms.

Senior medical assistance must be sought immediately; this will initiate a cascade of reactions resulting in early specialist opinion and the accessing of secondary specialist services. This is of extreme importance as research has demonstrated a significant decrease in both the mortality and morbidity rates in patients who are referred directly to specialist stroke services/units following CVA (DoH 2001a).

The patient requires a full neurological assessment commencing with the recording of a baseline GCS. The baseline neurological assessment will include recording the size, shape and reactivity of the patient's pupils, as subtle early warning signs may be present (Chapter 8). Risk factors for CVA development can be separated into non-modifiable and modifiable as defined in Box 10.2.

Box 10.2 High-risk factors for CVA development

- **Non-modifiable** risk factors include: age, race, ethnicity, sex, history of migraine headaches, sickle cell disease, previous history of transient ischaemic attacks (TIA), carotid artery stenosis, and possible heredity influences.
- **Modifiable** risk factors include: hypertension (prime importance), cardiac disease, atrial fibrillation, diabetes mellitus, hypercholesterolaemia, lifestyle choices: excessive alcohol intake, smoking, stimulant use, obesity, physical inactivity and oral contraceptive use.

Chapter 3 focused on cardiac emergencies and identified the close relationship between an altered cardiac physiology and the significantly increased potential for clot formation and a cerebral infarction. Thrombus formation due to an atherosclerotic plaque is not confined to the coronary arteries; other common areas include the mesenteric artery, resulting in an ischaemic bowel, and the carotid arteries supplying the brain. The areas of atheroma within the walls of the arteries lead to a weakened and stretched vessel. The end result of either an ischaemic event caused by an embolus or thrombus, or the rupture of a weakened vessel causing haemorrhage, is a reduction in both oxygen and nutrients to part of the brain, resulting in varying degrees of localized necrosis. An increased ICP may ensue, resulting in further necrosis and ultimately increased mortality and morbidity rates. The associated physical impact includes dysphasia, hemiplegia or paralyses affecting one side of the body, reduced cognition and a loss of the ability to swallow, particularly thin fluids resulting in aspiration pneumonia. CVA or stroke, as it is more commonly known, is a seriously debilitating illness.

Prevalence

In the UK 67,000 individuals will die of a stroke every year (BHF 2006). In comparison to AMI, the long-term physical and psychological consequences associated with a stroke can be seriously debilitating

The National Service Framework (NSF) for older people (DoH 2001a) identifies specific standards of care for those experiencing strokes. Although strokes are not confined to the older population, they are by far the majority of sufferers (ASA 2006). The American Stroke Association (ASA) (2006) states that each year 700,000 people experience a stroke, and of these 200,000 are recurrent attacks. In both the UK and the USA individuals of Afro-Caribbean heritage are twice as likely as Caucasians to experience a stroke. Stroke is the third leading cause of death in the USA and second within the UK (AHA 2006; ONS 2006), with 20–5 per cent of all acute hospital beds occupied by suffers (NAO 2005).

Around 88 per cent of strokes are ischaemic, while haemorrhagic stroke accounts for the other 12 per cent, of which 9 per cent are intracerebral and 3 per cent subarachnoid. The associated mortality rates are greatly related to the affected area of the brain, with the death rate from a subarachnoid or intracerebral haemorrhage exceeding 60 per cent (ASA 2006).

In the UK, over 300,000 individuals are living with various disabilities due to the aftermath of experiencing a CVA. International and national targets have been identified to prevent both the disease processes that integrate to cause CVA, and to minimalize the debilitating consequences of CVA once it has occurred. Despite several strategies, the immediate emergency care management of patients experiencing a CVA is poor with many emergency departments having no established plan of care or care pathway.

The contribution emergency clinicians can make to the long-term prognosis of patients who have suffered a CVA should not be underestimated. In the UK the current medical management of CVA centres on preventative medicine, with the prescribing of aspirin, statins and anti-hypertensive medications escalating at an alarming rate. Once an individual has experienced a CVA, the immediate medical management is varied; this is dependent on identifying the origin of the insult. Aspirin or anti-platelet agents have traditionally been the main form of treatment for non-haemorrhagic events. Many emergency departments are currently conducting trials aimed at delivering thrombolytic agents for ischaemic stroke, which has had a conditional licence for use since 2003. For thrombolysis to be effective, the agent has to be delivered within three hours of the event, this is reliant on a fast and accurate working diagnosis, the availability of CT scanning to confirm an ischaemic event, and patients meeting a strict entry criteria (to prevent cerebral haemorrhage), early trials have presented good results (AHA 2006). It is estimated that over 40 per cent of stroke patients have high blood glucose levels which are believed to be detrimental to the brain repair proceess due to glucose being converted to lactid acid in the face of hypoxia. Current research, funded by the Stroke Association, is directed at aggressively normalizing post-CVA blood glucose levels by administering insulin regimens. The essential care that all emergency clinicians can implement is outlined in Box 10.3.

The Royal College of Physicians (RCP 2004) recommends that if subarachnoid haemorrhage is suspected, and the patient presents with a decrease in their level of consciousness, an immediate CT scan is indicated. If there is not a decrease in the level of consciousness, the CT scan should be obtained within 12 hours. In both cases the results should be discussed with a neurosurgeon immediately (RCP 2004). It is well documented that neurosurgical

---

Box 10.3   The immediate care for those experiencing a CVA

Assess for actual or potential airway obstruction. A decrease in the level of consciousness can lead to the individual failing to maintain airway integrity. The assessment should focus on the look, listen and feel approach.

- *Look* for insufficient ventilation, use of the accessory muscles of breathing and cyanosis.
- *Listen* for gurgling, which indicates liquid substances within the upper airway. Snoring should alert the clinician that the tongue or soft tissues might be obstructing the airway: resolve this by placing the patient in the recovery position or applying either the head tilt, chin lift manoeuvre if the patient is insentient. Early referral to a specialist may prove vital.
- *Feel* for inadequate chest rise or airflow at the nose and mouth.

All CVA patients should receive supplementary oxygen, and this may need to be delivered via nasal cannula as patients are frequently hypoxic and confused and may misplace an oxygen mask. The inability to coordinate movement post-CVA places the individual at severe risk of the complications associated with immobility. If able, the patient's posture should be supported with pillows allowing for full chest expansion and the correction of paralysed areas preventing pressure sore development and maintaining dignity. Sitting patients upright has major physiological benefits; first, gravitational forces will allow swelling within the skull to drain, thus aiding the attenuation of an increased ICP and, second and most importantly, preventing patients from lying flat on their back will directly reduce the development of pneumonia. Patients must be made nil by mouth (NBM), until a risk assessment of their ability to swallow without aspirating water or food particles into their lungs is undertaken. While the patient is nil by mouth, they will require intravenous fluids containing glucose to help the brain repair, this is essential in the early stages. The patient's blood glucose, arterial oxygen level and hydration status should be closely monitored and normalized. DVT and PE prevention are vital and the patient should be mobilized as early as possible (RCP 2004).

---

referral rates for patients above 65 years of age are lower when compared to patients under 65, although there is no significant difference between age groups in the incidence of neurosurgical interventions in patients who are transferred (Munro et al. 2002). Many older patients, therefore, suffer increasing rates of mortality and morbidity due to the subjective beliefs of acute care clinicians.

When a bleed is confirmed, secondary brain injury can be prevented by the administration of Nimodipine, which can be administered via a nasogastric tube if the patient is unable to swallow. Nimodipine can prevent arterial spasm, thus allowing the bleed to clot. Further care follows the same route of secondary prevention as ischaemic stroke. In other words, provide supplementary oxygenation, maintain hydration and administer analgesia if necessary. The initial period spent within the emergency department can be very distressing for the patient and their relatives. Care should focus on preventing secondary brain injury, minimizing secondary complications due to immobility and expediting transfer to a specialist stroke unit or interventional service. The psychosocial impact on the patient and their relatives should not be underestimated: clinicians should try to relieve anxiety in both the patient and their relatives by providing support and information during this period.

Sickle cell disease

> **Scenario 10.2** Sickle cell crisis
>
> Richard Johns, a 27-year-old male, calls an ambulance after experiencing severe abdominal pain for the last hour. He has taken dihydrocodeine, which he is prescribed by his GP for his regular acute attacks of sickle cell pain. The pain has intensified and he is sweating profusely.
>
> He is able to talk, although he is obviously in pain. His respiratory rate is 27, regular, bi-laterally shallow. There are no signs of central or peripheral cyanosis. His radial pulse is weak, regular and recorded as 127 bpm, this is in conjunction with a CRT of 3 seconds. His blood pressure is recorded as 148/89. Mr Johns appears frightened and is pale. He adopts the foetal position and guards his abdomen, which is soft to touch. Although he is becoming increasingly annoyed at the number of questions being asked, his replies are rational, he is alert and orientated. His pupils are of equal size, recorded as 4mm, and reactive to light. He feels hot at both a peripheral, and central level.
>
> He has no known allergies and a past medical history of sickle cell disease.

D *Data* (scientific facts): Mr Johns appears to be demonstrating the early stages of compensatory shock, identified by the rapid respiratory rate. His radial pulse is weak, indicating a possible insult to the circulating volume, confirmed by the reduced CRT. His blood pressure is artificially elevated by the internal release of compensatory mediators (the sympathetic response). An oxygen saturation probe and cardiac monitoring should be employed in conjunction with a 12-lead ECG. Mr Johns is demonstrating many clinical signs associated with a possible ischaemic event in his abdomen, making this presentation potentially life-threatening. His sweaty, pale and clammy appearance may be due to the pain or the pathological alterations taking place within him. The clinician should understand that a patient exhibiting extreme pain is

---

Box 10.4 Causes of abdominal pain

- Irritation of nerves
- Inflammation of the peritoneum
- Irritation/inflammation of mucosa
- Direct organ irritation/inflammation/ischaemia
- Musculature spasm/contraction

---

always a cause for concern, due to the altered physiology that is associated with pain development. Box 10.4 outlines the physiological causes of abdominal pain (Chapter 7).

E *Emotions* (intuition): Mr Johns suffers from a chronic history of sickle cell disease. This places him at increased risk of vaso-occlusive, haematological and infectious processes, all of which can be extremely painful and lead to organ failure and death. The clinician will intuitively take this presentation seriously due to the patient's appearance, commencing early interventional therapy. Care will be expedited by placing the patient in a high dependency area, with the negation of serious illness the priority.

A *Advantages*: as with all potentially critically ill patients, high-flow oxygen should be commenced via a reservoir bag and mask. Intravenous access should be obtained as early into the presentation as possible as sickle cell presentations commonly involve dehydration and the associated decrease in peripheral circulation, precipitating the red blood cells to sludge. Routine bloods should be obtained, including inflammatory tests and cross-matching, in case of severe anaemia, as a blood transfusion may be necessary. Analgesia should be a priority and all progressive emergency departments will have a set protocol to follow. This protocol should be based on the World Health Organization step approach to analgesia (WHO 1996). There are many pain assessment scales available, and it is recommended that emergency clinicians use a minimalist approach due to the clinical symptoms. Table 10.1 demonstrates an example.

Table 10.1 Categorical rating scale for acute pain

Pain Score	Appropriate analgesia
0 = No pain	N/A
1 = Mild pain	Non-opioids
2 = Moderate pain	Weak opioids combinations
3 = Severe pain	Stronger opioid combination
4 = Very severe pain	Opioids titrated to pain

This assessment scale directly relates to the choice of analgesia, which reduces the subjective opinions of clinicians. As with the assessment of all patients in pain, the objective findings such as those associated with the sympathetic response should be included.

Obtaining a thorough presenting and past medical history can reveal instigators to the current circumstances. Patients experiencing a sickle cell crisis often present with a similar clinical presentation to an acute abdomen, although once appropriate treatment commences, many of the comparable signs dissipate.

D *Disadvantages* (**differential diagnosis**): when faced with a patient presenting with a relevant medical history the assessing practitioner should not make assumptions that an exacerbation of a chronic condition has led to the current presentation. This presentation may be due to an acute abdomen and this possibility should be negated, which is of particular importance in this case as the patient may be exhibiting signs of hypovolaemic shock. The pain could also be due to less sinister pathologies such as a urinary tract infection or chronic constipation resulting from the use of opioids.

Definition and prevalence

Sickle cell disease is a genetically inherited disorder whereby the suffer inherits two variant haemoglobin genes, one from each parent. It mainly affects individuals of Afro-Caribbean heritage, although similar genetic pathologies exist within Mediterranean countries and the Middle East. The high incidence of the sickle cell gene in these regions of the world is due to the sickle cell's ability to make red blood cells resistant to the malaria parasite (Clancy and McVicar 2002). Individuals who inherit just a single variant gene are referred to as having sickle cell trait, these healthy carriers are protected against malaria and do not develop sickle cell disease. Those who inherit both copies of the gene develop sickle cell disease and are not protected from malaria. Thirty years ago the life expectancy of an individual experiencing sickle cell disease was around 14 years, today with modern treatments it exceeds 50 years of age (Claster and Vichinsky 2003). It is estimated that there are in excess of 15,000 individuals living with sickle cell or haemoglobinopathies within the UK (Anionwu and Atkin 2001).

Pathophysiology

Sickle cell disease occurs from genetic abnormalities in haemoglobin construction where a single amino acid substitution creates a cascade of events leading to the deformation of an essential component of red blood cells. The red blood cells become misshapen, rigid and sticky, resembling a sickle (Figure 10.1). This sickling leads to an increase in blood viscosity; RBCs can adhere to the inner layer of arterial walls and literally get stuck while travelling through the

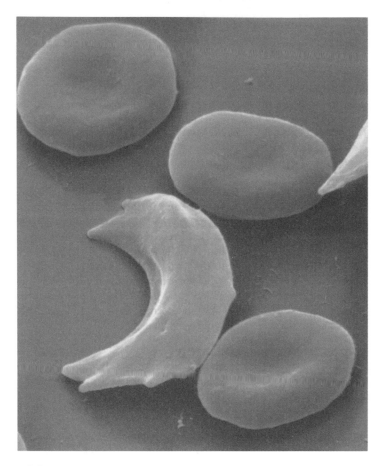

Source: Saladin (2005)

Figure 10.1 Sickle cell disease

capillaries. Blood flow becomes obstructed, depriving tissues and organs of oxygen and nutrients. In the acute phase cellular hypoxia can cause severe pain referred to as the sickle cell crisis. Excessive intracellular acidity and the abnormal shape of the sickled cells also cause water and potassium loss resulting in dehydration. Sickle cells also have a shorter life span (10 to 20 days) compared to that of normal red blood cells (90 to 120 days). Although the body compensates for the decrease in viable red blood cells, the overall red blood cell count diminishes, resulting in anaemia, hence the term sickle cell anaemia. Common triggers include hypoxia, infection and dehydration.

With repeated attacks a chronic and progressive destruction to the internal tissues and organs occurs. Commonly affected areas include the spleen, lungs and liver.

Acute chest syndrome occurs when the lungs are deprived of oxygen during a crisis, it can be very painful, dangerous and potentially life-threatening. This is a leading cause of acute presentation among sickle cell patients and is the most common cause of death, with an extensive stroke being the second (Gladwin et al. 1999).

Treatment

Treatment initially centres on pain control, supplementary oxygenation and rehydration. The first 20 minutes of care can be structured by adopting the NIH and NHLBI (2002) treatment algorithm (Figure 10.2), this will provide novice practitioners with a plan of initial care and expedite treatment for suffers. The identification of the cause then signals the implementation of definitive care.

Pulmonary embolism

Scenario 10.3 Pulmonary embolism

Mrs Boyer is a 33-year-old female who collapsed after leaving the arrivals section of Heathrow airport, following a long-haul flight from Cape Town. She is sweating profusely and complaining of shooting pains in her chest.

She is assessed by a rapid response paramedic who identifies the following:

1 Airway clear, patient able to talk.
2 Patient is breathing, although very short of breath. There are no signs of central cyanosis and her respiratory rate is recorded as 27. Pulse oximetry reveals SpO2 88% on 28% oxygen. On auscultation, air entry sounds normal although the patient's breathing is very shallow. The patient states that she has a severe stabbing pain in her chest which increases on inspiration.
3 Patient has a bounding radial pulse that is regular and recorded as 124bpm. CRT is recorded as 4 seconds. The initial blood pressure is 90/54.
4 Although Mrs Boyer is extremely anxious, her AVPU is A.
5 No visible signs of injury, and the patient feels warm to touch.

Mrs Boyer has no known allergies; she has no relevant medical history, although she smokes and takes the oral contraceptive.

D *Data* (scientific facts): when a patient presents sweating profusely, in combination with a rapid respiratory rate, bounding and rapid pulse, and a reduced CRT, the clinical indicators of a severe illness are all too apparent. The tachycardia and tachypnoea indicate the compensatory phase of shock,

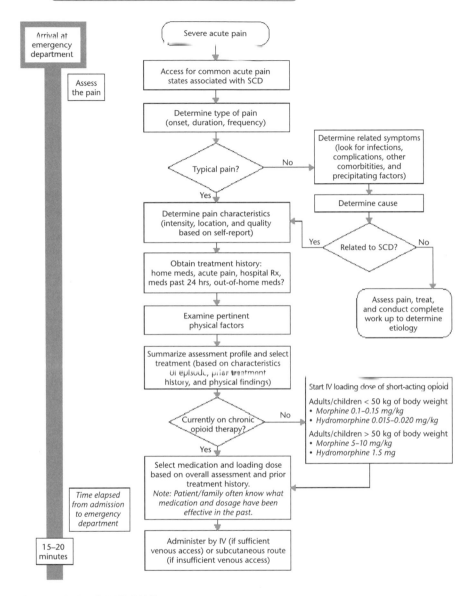

Source: NIH and NHLBI (2002)

Figure 10.2 The management of sickle cell disease

the oxygen saturation level is life-threatening, the slightly reduced blood pressure indicates the beginning of decompensatory shock and haemodynamic collapse. If this condition is left untreated, the patient is at great risk of impending cardiac arrest.

E *Emotions* (intuition): the physical presentation, when combined with the presenting history, signals the realistic possibility of a pulmonary embolism. Recent air travel in conjunction with several established high risk factors for clot development, such as smoking and the contraceptive pill, reinforce this developing working diagnosis. The patient will be treated within the resuscitation room and specialist assistance requested, including an anaesthetist as the oxygen desaturation may lead to imminent arrest. Presentations of PE are varied depending on the extent to which the blood flow has been curtailed; extensive vessel occlusion commonly results in patients presenting in a moribund state. The classic clinical signs associated with PE centre on pleuritic chest pain, shortness of breath, tachypnoea, tachycardia, and possibly haemoptysis.

A *Advantages*: the immediate application of high-flow oxygen and specialist referral may save this patient's life. A baseline arterial blood gas should be ascertained; in many cases the administration of high-flow oxygen will resolve the hypoxaemia and symptoms may lessen, pulse oximetry should be continually monitored, in combination with the patient's level of consciousness. Intravenous access should be obtained as soon as possible as the impending haemodynamic collapse will make it virtually impossible to gain peripheral access. Intravenous morphine is the analgesic of choice; this should be titrated to the patient's response and vital signs. Bloods should be sent for routine examination and for specialist tests, these might include D-dimer if the patient meets local inclusion criteria (Box 10.5). The patient must be placed on a cardiac monitor and an ECG obtained. The ECG may reveal strain to the right side of the heart although results are not solely diagnostic. Continual ECG monitoring is vital due to the distinct possibility of arrhythmia development. The previous diagnostic tool of choice was the ventilation/perfusion or V/Q scan which has been superseded by the use of computerized tomographic pulmonary angiography (CTPA). Although this test may reveal a positive diagnosis, patients presenting in a compromised fashion may need treatment prior to transfer, to stabilize their condition.

The British Thoracic Society (BTS 2003) has extensively researched the evidence base underpinning PE, which has resulted in the publication of specific guidelines that now underpin current clinical practice.

In suspected PE, with circulatory collapse, thrombolysis is the treatment of choice (BTS 2003); therapy should be commenced as soon as possible, once contraindications have been considered. In patients presenting with severe symptoms associated with PE, but no circulatory collapse, heparin is recommended due to the decreased association with major haemorrhage.

D *Disadvantages* (differential diagnosis): chest pain with a shortness of breath is a common presentation, but identifying that the origin of the presentation is a complicated and laborious process. The immediate focus of the assessor has been discussed but there is a potential for the cause of the presentation or

Box 10.5   Management of suspected non-massive pulmonary embolism

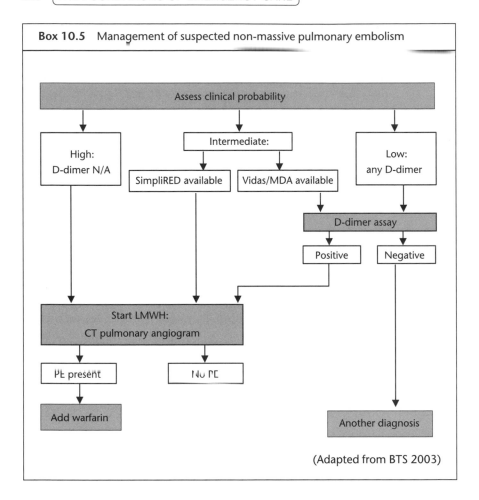

(Adapted from BTS 2003)

pathology to be a symptom of several other disease processes. The primary disease to negate is an acute coronary syndrome; other common presentations include chest infections, pleurisy and hysterical hyperventilation.

Prevalence

The BTS (2003) states that half the incidence of VTE formation develops while patients are in hospital or care settings, with an associated mortality rate of 10 per cent, making prevention tactics a priority. PE is a major cause of death with an estimated annual death rate ranging between 2.4–6 per cent per 100,000 in the United States (Lilienfeld 2000). As with coronary vascular disease, there is a significant difference between Caucasians and people of Afro-Caribbean heritage who have nearly three times the death rate. Seventy per cent of patients experiencing a PE have an associated deep vein thrombosis; therefore the initial assessment should include an inspection and measurement of the patient's calf area. It has been identified, however, that the aetiology of many of the serious or massive pulmonary emboli originate within the larger vessels of the thigh, therefore limiting the effectiveness of calf assessment.

Pathophysiology

Most PEs derive from a thrombus that has formed within the legs; the clot dislodges and becomes an embolus. This 'clot on the trot' is forced through the circulation until it encounters an area of narrowed vessels; this is commonly within the distal regions of the pulmonary artery. If the embolus is particularly large, it may clot proximally within the lung causing a massive obstruction to the distal areas of the lung circulation, thus, causing a severe perfusion ventilation mismatch.

Preventative measures

Patients should be encouraged to mobilize as soon as possible; anticipate DVT formation in patients when their mobility is compromised, by either the presenting problem or in those receiving treatment that will immobilize them, i.e. the application of a plaster of Paris. Other high-risk factors include previous DVT, increased blood viscosity and established clotting disorders. Patients at risk should be encouraged to keep hydrated, mobilize within their ability, including the flexion and extension of the feet, avoid lying with their legs crossed and, if at increased risk, prophylactic low molecular weight heparin should be commenced for the duration of their hospitalization.

Gastrointestinal haemorrhage

Scenario 10.4   Gastrointestinal bleed

Brian Taylor, a 27-year-old, presents with severe indigestion and collapses whist waiting to be seen. He vomits around 300mls of mixed fresh blood and clots onto the floor. He is coughing and states he had a similar episode one hour ago.

His respiratory rate is recorded as 29 with full chest expansion. Pulse oximetry reveals an oxygen saturation of 96 per cent before oxygen therapy is commenced. His radial pulse is weak and only just palpable, the rhythm is regular and recorded as134bpm. CRT is recorded as three seconds. The initial blood pressure is 82/54. Post-vomiting the patient looks pale and clammy. He is alert although it requires repeated questioning to ascertain a response. He feels cold to the touch and his auxiliary temperature is recorded as 35.5

He has no medical history but regularly takes non-steroidal anti-inflammatory drugs, smokes 20–30 cigarettes per day and states he binge drinks alcohol at the weekends.

D *Data* (scientific facts): the recorded data and clinical presentation indicate an ominous presentation; an upper gastrointestinal (GI) bleed. Although the patient is able to talk, his airway is at risk from the aspiration of vomit or blood and from a potential decrease in his level of consciousness. The respiratory rate demonstrates compensation for the inadequate circulation, which is confirmed by the reduced CRT, the weak and barely palpable pulse, and the decompensated blood pressure. Due to the nature of the illness this patient may also have established anaemia due to degeneration of the gut lining over a period of time. The combination of tachypnoea, tachycardia and hypotension are indicative of decompensatory shock. The patient may also be demonstrating the early signs of inadequate cerebral oxygenation; indicated by a lack of cognition.

E *Emotions* (intuition): the experienced clinician will know that GI bleeds commonly result in cardiac arrest due to hypovolaemia and will, therefore, treat this presentation with utmost urgency. This will involve the immediate transferral of the patient to the resuscitation room and the call for expert senior assistance. The experienced clinician will attach the patient to monitoring equipment and commence regular recording and evaluation of the patient's vital signs. Essential equipment will be checked for viability and this should include suction, which may prove vital.

A *Advantages*: the application of immediate high-flow oxygen, senior assistance and the insertion of two wide bore cannula are essential, bloods should be taken and fluids commenced. Suddenly increasing the arterial pressure may be detrimental to the patient due to the possibility of dislodging clotted areas and recommencing bleeding (popping the clot). The titration of fluids to maintain a systemic blood pressure of around 90mmHg or MAP of 60mmHg is therefore recommended; alternatives include using 200ml fluid infusions to maintain the blood pressure. When a patient is actively bleeding, fluid replacement is essential to maintain an adequate circulation but, if the patient is actively losing blood, then blood is the choice for fluid replacement. If the presentation wasn't severe and the blood pressure was stable, a postural blood pressure would be indicated as this could help to identify the early establishment of shock. The patient will require a urinary catheter and the insertion of a CVP line to monitor fluid resuscitation. There are several initial treatment options for patients experiencing a GI bleed; these are discussed later.

Table 10.2 Common causes of gastrointestinal haemorrhage

Diagnosis	Approximate %
Peptic ulcer	35–50
Gastroduodenal erosions	8–15
Oesophagitis	5–15
Varices	5–10

(Adapted from the BSGEC, 2002.)

D *Disadvantages* (**differential diagnosis**): an early diagnosis is essential to the subsequent treatment of GI bleeding, as there are several possible causes (Table 10.2). If the cause is related to alcoholism, liver cirrhosis and the development of oesophageal varices, the prognosis is significantly worse than for the erosion of a gastric ulcer (Dallal and Palmer 2001). The mortality rate for oesophageal varices is around 50 per cent (Gow and Chapman 2001).

A comprehensive history is essential, although, when faced by a patient presenting in an already compromised state, emergency treatment is indicated.

Epigastric pain, and heartburn or dysphagia are common presentations among young patients, the presenting history will usually include the recent consumption of alcohol. For younger patients gastric ulceration is the most likely cause of upper GI bleeds, for older patients, over 45 years of age, a risk assessment and liberal use of investigative endoscopy to negate stomach cancer are reasonable (BSG 2006).

Prevalence

Gastrointestinal bleeding is a common medical emergency with an estimated incidence ranging from 50–150 per 100,000 of the population per year, resulting in an annual cost to the NHS of £1.4 billion. There is a direct correlation between lower socio-economic groups and the development of GI bleeding (BSGEC 2002). According to the British Society of Gastroenterology (2002), upper GI bleeds are most commonly associated with peptic ulcer formation (Table 10.2) due either to long-term non-steroidal anti-inflammatory drug (NSAIDs) use, Helicobacter pylori colonization of the stomach or excessive alcohol consumption.

Treatment

The patient will need to be stabilized within the emergency department, depending on the severity of the bleeding and the effect this has on the patient (a GI bleed may exacerbate other pathologies). This will be centred on the

ABCDE approach and problems addressed as they are encountered, this may include intubation, fluid resuscitation and the administration of a pressor agent. Once stabilized, the patient should be transferred to an area where there are appropriately trained staff or an area of high dependency nursing. The BSG guidelines for upper GI haemorrhage include an algorithm for the management of patients (page iv of the guidelines). The algorithm consists of two distinct but interchangeable pathways. The guidance indicates the immediate transfer of patients to an endoscopy facility in the presence of a major GI bleed, although this is clearly in the patient's best interest, it may not be current practice in many areas.

The acute treatment for an active GI bleed is often dependent on the level of skill of the clinicians the patient encounters. The BSG recommend that emergency interventional endoscopy is the treatment of choice for patients with upper gastrointestinal haemorrhage. A skilled practitioner can, first, directly visualize/identify the actual disease process and the amount of localized damage and, second, deliver definitive treatment. All hospitals should offer a 24-hour emergency endoscopy service as this has the potential to save lives by reducing morbidity, and in the long term will prove to be cost effective (BSG 2006).

Preventative measures

The BSG estimates that 40 per cent of the population will at some time experience symptoms related to acid reflux, dyspepsia or gastric ulcer formation. It is therefore recommended that clinicians identify early warning signs and that preventative measures are taken (BSG 2006). Patients should be advised to avoid known precipitants they associate with their dyspepsia in order to prevent deterioration and reoccurrence. These include smoking, alcohol, coffee, chocolate, fatty foods and being overweight (NICE 2004a).

Diabetes

Scenario 10.5 Diabetic ketoacidosis
Mohammed Azad, a 62-year-old of Asian origin, arrives by ambulance after collapsing at home 30 minutes ago. His son accompanies him. On presentation he is able to talk, although he speaks little English; he sounds very dry and appears slightly pale, his son, who is present, states his father is talking gibberish and that this is very different to how he normally behaves. His father has not been his usual self for a few weeks and has been feeling very tired during this period.

Mr Azad's respiratory rate is 30, regular and shallow. His radial pulse is 121 strong and regular, CRT > 2 seconds. Blood pressure is 148/96. Mr Azad looks slightly pale and very dehydrated. His skin appears dry with skin flaking off and although he utters incomprehensible sounds, his mouth is extremely dry. His GCS is recorded as E4 V3 M5 = 12/15.

There are no visible injuries and his temperature is recorded as 37.9. He has no known medical history.

D *Data* (scientific facts): Mr Azad's presentation is complex and contains many pathological possibilities; this therefore makes the structuring of his care paramount, as significant data may be missed.

Initially Mr Azad is able to talk but appears to be presenting with an acute confusional state (Box 10.6). There are many potential causes for this presentation and they will be considered in combination with other prominent points of the patient assessment.

Mr Azad's respiratory rate indicates hyperventilation and either a respiratory problem or respiratory compensation for another underlying problem. Supplementary oxygen should be commenced and a pulse oximeter attached, chest auscultation may identify an underlying cause. His pulse is regular and strong but tachycardic, this is combined with a reduced capillary refill time and a slightly raised blood pressure. All elderly patients presenting with a reduced level of consciousness should have a baseline Glasgow coma score recorded. The presenting history, in combination with his pyrexia, will prompt the requisition of several tests to begin the negation process.

E *Emotions* (intuition): many patients attend due to multiple pathologies, particularly the elderly. An experienced clinician will recognize the many risk factors for serious illness, and commence a plan of care aimed at eliminating the most serious or life-threatening first. These include a significant cardiovascular event like CVA or AMI or hypoxaemia and an infective cause.

A *Advantages*: as with all patients presenting with potentially serious symptoms, the immediate application of high-flow oxygen may prevent further deterioration. Senior assistance should be sought and a cascade of data collection commenced. Mr Azad will be attached to a cardiac monitor and a 12-lead ECG recorded. Intravenous access is paramount, blood tests will include a full blood count as anaemia and an infective process may be a probable cause, urea and electrolytes as dehydration has been clinically diagnosed. This will include an overview of his renal and hepatic function. Cardiac-specific enzymes, blood cultures and a blood glucose analysis will be necessary as this presentation has all the trademarks of hyperglycaemia. A baseline arterial blood gas should be ascertained; this may identify hypoxaemia, hypercapnia or a metabolic acidosis, all of which are possible with this type of presentation.

Although the patient appears dry, fluid administration should only be commenced once the patient has had a senior member auscultate his lungs for possible pulmonary oedema, as heart failure is possible and fluids may exacerbate the presentation; a chest X-ray will also assist in excluding other pathologies such as pneumonia.

Mr Azad's AVPU score is currently A; neurological observations such be commenced as they may provide an early indicator of a deterioration in his clinical state. An infective cause is highly likely despite the absence of a severely elevated temperature, therefore a source of infection should be negated. An appropriately trained clinician will undertake further in-depth neurological assessment as a TIA or CVA (Scenario 10.1) could be a cause.

D *Disadvantages* (**differential diagnosis**): when confronted by an elderly patient demonstrating a reduced level of consciousness or confusion, an inexperienced clinician may generalize and associate the condition with chronic dementia, this should only be concluded when those close to the patient or his GP confirm it. In this case his son clearly states the confusion is acute and therefore instigating pathologies should be eliminated. Prime causes include:

- TIA/CVA
- Sepsis and infective causes
- Alcohol or drug intoxication (can be iatrogenic)
- Organ failure (renal)
- Metabolic disorders (diabetes)
- Blood oxygen mismatches (MI/PE)
- Constipation and urine infections.

Acute confusional states

Box 10.6 Assessment of acute confusional states

It is estimated that around 30 per cent of acute medical presentations are associated with confusion. An acute confusional state can be defined as a sudden state of severe confusion and rapid changes in brain function; clinically the patient is inaccessible to normal contact. Symptoms may include an inability to concentrate and disorganized thinking. Rambling, irrelevant or incoherent speech, impaired short-term memory, disorientation and an impaired level of consciousness demonstrate this clinical manifestation. A mini-mental state examination is frequently undertaken as part of the assessment.

(Ramrakha and Moore 2004)

Hyperglycaemia

In the case of Mr Azad, hyperglycaemia was confirmed by a simple fingerprick examination of his blood on a glucometor. This routine test can be vital in identifying the patient with undiagnosed diabetes mellitus. It is extremely cost effective and user friendly, it cannot, however, be used to diagnose diabetes. The early identification of those at risk of this disease process can limit the devastating damage which results due to its insidious development. If left undiagnosed, as in the case of Mr Azad, until the level of glucose or sugar in his blood reaches such a high level that he becomes confused via clinical dehydration, vast internal damage will have already occurred (Box 10.7) (WHO 1999).

Box 10.7   Internal damage associated with diabetes mellitus

- Thickening of capillary membranes leads to retina and glomerular compromise.
- Accelerated atherosclerotic deposits via hyperlipidaemia associated with hyperglycaemia.
- Neuropathic and cardiovascular compromise instigates decreased sensation and a reduced distal blood supply resulting in arterial insufficiency, ulceration and ischaemic changes particularly evident in the feet (diabetic foot ulcers).
- Increased susceptibility to infection resulting from a compromise of the immune system.

Definition and prevalence

Diabetes mellitus is a disorder affecting the metabolism of carbohydrates (sugars) resulting from a deficiency or a resistance to insulin, characterized by increasing levels of sugar in the blood, commonly described in two similar, but distinct formats (Box 10.8). The Department of Health state that there are at least 2.3 million diabetics in England alone and the number is set to escalate, primarily due to the increasing numbers of clinical obseity; 34 per cent of females in England are clinically obese which means they are 13 times more likely to develop Type 2 diabetes (DoH 2006), more worryingly, childhood obesity is leading to Type 2 diabetes in early life (DoH 2001b). This form of diabetes has a particularly high rate of associated morbidity and mortality. The aetiology of Type 2 diabetes mellitus is multifactorial, involving a genetic predisposition; it also has strong behavioural or lifestyle components. This

---

Box 10.8 Presentation classification and pathophysiology

Type 1 Insulin-Dependent Diabetes

- Sudden destruction of insulin-secreting cells leads to acute hyperglycaemic episode characterized by insulin deficiency and ketosis resulting in gastric stasis, coma and death if left untreated
- Accounts for 10–15% of cases (DoH 2001b)
- Results early in life as a consequence of an autoimmune reaction (presentation < 25) with destruction of pancreatic islet beta-cells
- Daily insulin injections needed to sustain life
- Insulin requirements, physical levels of activity and diet need correlation
- Potential for hypoglycaemia high
- Can be idiopathic
- Life expectancy reduced on average by 20 years

Type 2 Non-Insulin-Dependent Diabetes

- Insidious onset characterized by increasingly defective ability to secrete and utilize insulin. Eventually leading to hyperglycaemia
- Not traditionally associated with ketosis, results in many associated disease processes being present when disease is first diagnosed
- Accounts for 85 per cent of cases (DoH 2001b)
- Tradionally associated with middle-age onset (> 40)
- Increasing teenage/young adult onset: direct correlation with increasing levels of obesity (DoH 2001b)
- Considered a preventible disease
- Commonly associated with high fat/calorie diet, lack of exercise and obesity (ADA 2005)
- In many cases diet and lifestyle modification may curtail symptoms and disease establishment
- Life expectancy reduced by 10 years (dependent on age of onset)

Prolonged exposure to hyperglycaemia causes widespread tissue damage, commonly affected areas include the eyes, kidneys and feet. Diabetes is the leading cause of renal failure and blindness (in working age) and the second commonest cause of limb amputation.

Diabetes accounts for 5 per cent of the total NHS resources; it is estimated that 10 per cent of inpatient services are taken by those experiencing diabetes.

---

insidious form of diabetes is up to six times as prevalent in people from South Asian backgrounds, and three and a half times in those with an Afro-Caribbean heritage. There is also a disproportionately high association with lower social classes (DoH 2001b). The American Diabetes Association (2005) estimates that a third of individuals with Type 2 diabetes are undiagnosed.

The National Service Framework for Diabetes

The National Service Framework (NSF) for Diabetes (DoH 2001b) sets standards in relation to both the prevention and management of diabetes. These standards are predominately directed at Type 2 diabetes as the majority of cases are preventable.

Diagnosis

Due to the potential legal and medical implications associated with the diagnosis of diabetes, the World Health Organization (WHO) have stated the diagnosis of diabetes must be confirmed by the analysis of a fasting plasma glucose sample or whole blood sample. A diagnosis should never be made on a urine sample or a fingerprick sample alone.

The diagnosis is confirmed primarily by:

- a fasting sample > 7.0 (plasma sample)
- a random sample > 11.1 mmol/l.

The test must then be repeated on another day to confirm the diagnosis (WHO 1999). Those individuals that fall between the two figures are classified as high risk for the development of diabetes.

Acute diabetic emergencies: hyperglycaemia

Diabetic ketoacidosis, hyperosmolar non-ketotic syndrome and lactic acidosis are the three serious acute complications of diabetes, although hypoglycaemia is also a common occurrence, more prevalent in those requiring insulin.

Type 1 diabetic ketoacidosis (DKA)

DKA is a potentially life-threatening complication of diabetes resulting from an inadequate concentration of insulin in the blood. Cells are unable to utilize glucose in the absence of insulin, resulting in a reliance on stored body fat for energy. Both blood glucose levels and the by-products of fat metabolism, known as ketone bodies, esculate. The internal environment becomes increasingly acidotic with both the respiratory and renal sytems working to maintain homeostasis.

DKA is responsible for around 80 per cent of all deaths in children with diabetes, with cerebral oedema being the direct cause of death in the majority of cases (DoH 2005). It is usually due to poor insulin management, co-existing disease or first occurrence.

Initial treatment centres on administration of oxygen, aggressive rehydration and insulin therapy (Box 10.9).

Box 10.9   Treatment of diabetic ketoacidosis

- High-flow oxygen administration – early intubation if indicated.
- Aggressive rehydration – refer to local guidelines (beware of co-existing cardiac disease).
- Early measurements of central venous pressure in those with, or at risk of, cardiac disease.
- Potassium replacement titrated to arterial blood gas analysis.
- Insulin replacement (sliding scale titrated to blood glucose level which should remain at 10–14mmol/L for the first 24 hours, 5 per cent glucose may be necessary).
- The regular monitoring/assessment of the patient is essential.
- Early identification of cerebral oedema is vital (severe headaches and drowsiness are cardinal symptoms).
- Due to gastric stasis – patient nil by mouth.
- Urinary catheterization and a nasogastric tube will be necessary in those demonstrating oliguria or a decreased level of consciousness.
- The use of sodium barcabionate remains controversal and is only indicated in severe metabolic acidosis (pH < 7.0).

(Based on Ramrakha and Moore 2004)

Type 2 Hyperosmolar non-ketotic syndrome (HONK)

Usually the first presentation of Type 2 diabetes (> 30 per cent), the patient will display symptoms highlighted in Table 10.3.

The patient can appear extremely dehydrated (as in the case of Mr Azad) and have a reduced level of consciousness. It is estimated that the mortality rate from HONK exceeds 50 per cent (DOH 2001b).

The management for DKA and HONK are similar with thromboembolism a serious consequence of both; therefore all patients should be risk assessed and prophylactic anticoagulation commenced. This is particularly important in Type 2 diabetics due to the increased blood viscosity through extreme

Table 10.3   Signs and symptoms of diabetes

Signs	Symptoms
• Urine infections and opportunist infections, i.e., thrush, mouth ulcers	• Intense/increased thirst
	• Polyuria
• Cataract development	• Lethargy
• Deteriorating vision (retinopathy)	• Paraesthesia in extremities
• Reduced circulation in the feet and foot ulcers	• Possible weight loss

---

Box 10.10   Treatment of HONK

- High-flow oxygen administration – early intubation if indicated.
- Gain immediate IV access.
- Rehydration – Ramrakha and Moore (2004) recommend central venous pressure monitoring in all presentations.
- Early anti-coagulation may prove life-saving.
- Insulin replacement (sliding scale titrated to blood glucose level).
- The regular monitoring/assessment of the patient is essential.
- Due to gastric stasis – patient nil by mouth.
- Urinary catheterization and a nasogastric tube will be necessary in those demonstrating oliguria or a decreased level of consciousness.

(Based on Ramrakha and Moore 2004)

---

hyperglycaemia and dehydration, both of which will make the blood stagnate and increase the likelyhood of clot development.

Traditionally DKA is a very uncommon presenting feature in Type 2 diabetes, but recent clinical studies have identified that around half of younger patients presenting with Type 2 diabetes also present with DKA (DoH 2006).

Box 10.11 demonstrates a synopsis of the management of hypoglycaemia, a consequence of both types of diabetes, when managed with medications that actively lower blood glucose levels.

Box 10.11   Treatment of hypoglycaemia

- Hypoglycaemia should be negated in all patients presenting with a decrease in their level of consciousness or collapse.
- The physical manifestation of hypoglycaemia commonly results when the blood glucose falls below 3.6mmol/l, with a direct correlation between the presenting symptoms and the decrease in blood glucose.
- Confusion, slurred speech and coma can occur with levels < 2.5mmol/l.
- If the patient is able to tolerate fluids, the oral administration of a sugary substance is indicated (Hypostop gel/dissolved sugar lumps).
- When the patient presentation includes a reduced level of consciousness and IV access is established, glucose 50 per cent can be titrated to effect (usually 25–50mls). Lower concentrations are used in children.
- Glucogon can be injected via the subcutaneous and intramuscular routes and is therefore indicated when no IV access has been established.
- Beware patients presenting with a normalized blood glucose following the earlier administration of glucogon. They can suddenly relapse when the effects wear off.

The care of the diabetic patient is not only based on their immediate physiological needs. The NSF for diabetes clearly identifies 12 standards, many of which relate to emergency care, these are highlighted in Table 10.4 which identifies how they can be applied to provide excellence in care for patients experiencing diabetes.

Diabetes is a lifelong condition and despite increasing knowledge and holistic programmes of care, hyperglycaemia remains a leading cause of morbidity and mortality throughout the world (English and Williams 2004). Forging a solid and trusting relationship with diabetics is essential to their long-term health outcomes.

Emergency care staff should opportunistically screen patients for the development of diabetes, and routinely risk assess known diabetics for the development of the serious associated complications previously stated.

Embodied in the NSF is the central value of the NHS Plan that good service is the outcome of genuine partnership between the patient and the provider.

Table 10.4 Providing excellence in care of diabetes

Standard	Application
Standards 1, 2 and 9: strategies to reduce and identify Type 2 diabetes	• Identification of those at high-risk of diabetes development (Box 10.8) • Liberal use of fingerprick blood analysis for possible hyperglycaemia • Regular interdepartmental health awareness and education campaigns
Standards 3, 4 and 10: patient empowerment and reduction of long-term complications	• Ownership of condition firmly placed with the individual • All patients attending with history of diabetes to have risk assessment undertaken on secondary disease development (primary care referral)
Standards 7 and 8: implementation of a rapid and effective treatment pathway for diabetic emergencies	• Implementation of a multi-agency fast track patient-focused protocol/care pathway including risk assessment for secondary complications • Pathways should be monitored at regular intervals for effectiveness, i.e expediating care
Standards 11 and 12: mulidisciplinary support	• A network of local services exist for support and long-term assistance; the patient should be made aware of the network and referred to appropriate services (a fast track referral system will benefit both emergency clinicians and the patient). GP made aware of contact and service provision

Self-harming

Scenario 10.6 Self-harming

Patrick Johnson attends after lacerating his forearm. He appears well; his respiratory rate is recorded as 14, pulse 72, blood pressure 124/72, and temperature 36.5.

The wounds are on the inner aspect of the forearm, and have stopped bleeding. The damage is minor with no distal neurovascular damage. The wounds are limited to the dermis with no subcutaneous tissue visible. The largest of the three wounds is approximately 4cm in length. There are several scars on both arms. When asked how the lacerations occurred, Mr Johnson states that he is under a lot of pressure and cuts himself with a Stanley blade. His further questioning reveals a chronic history of deliberate self-harm (DSH). This includes several drug overdoses including aspirin and paracetamol.

Past medical history includes depression after his wife left him. He currently takes anti-depressant medication. He has never been a psychiatric in-patient.

D *Data* (scientific facts): when confronted by a patient who has actively harmed himself, the practitioner needs to adopt a holistic approach to the assessment process, despite the initial data indicating limited physical damage, the risk potential for further DSH may be high. In addition, the practitioner will need to ascertain if Mr Johnson has taken an overdose, or is under the effects of drugs or alcohol.

The NICE (2004b) guidelines recommend that the triage process should include a preliminary psychosocial assessment, establishing the patient's willingness to remain for assessment/treatment, and their level of distress or mental illness (Box 10.12).

Box 10.12 The initial assessment of self-harm presentations

- Base initial assessment on ABCDE approach
- Early risk assessment is essential to establish possibility of lethal presentation, further harm, potential harm to others and of patient absconding
- The initial assessment should also identify previous mental illness and drug use
- The provision of a named point of contact may establish cooperation
- If mental capacity is diminished, or significant mental illness or risk potential identified, the patient should be prevented from leaving and urgent MH assistance sought

(Based on NICE 2004b guidelines)

E *Emotions* (intuition): DSH is a common presentation to EDs, experienced practitioners take the initial assessment seriously, as identifying the motive and the physical consequences are equally important. The patient should be cared for in an appropriate environment away from distressing stimuli.

A *Advantages*: further questioning should be directed at identifying a possible overdose, a baseline neurological assessment should be recorded, and venous access and bloods obtained, if an overdose is suspected. Within the first hour of many overdoses the administration of activated charcoal can minimize the absorption of the poison/medication; advice on the management of patients can be obtained from national poisons units and web-based sites such as TOX-BASE. The patient should be offered a named member of staff to liaise with and placed in a quiet area minimizing further distress, and this early interventional approach may prevent the patient from leaving and provide a positive atmosphere.

D *Disadvantages* (differential diagnosis): during the triage process the patient must be asked what their intentions are: do they, or did they, intend to kill themselves? If the answer is yes, or the patient is demonstrating signs of acute mental illness, the psychiatric liaison team should be called immediately and the department's security staff made aware of the patient. Other high-risk factors are identified in Box 10.13. Physical effects should also be assessed including the full assessment of the minor injuries in case underlying structures such as tendons or nerves have been damaged. The patient will require adequate analgesia prior to suturing if necessary.

Box 10.13 High-risk factors or behaviours

- Patient is having suicidal thoughts or demonstrating suicidal tendencies
- Previous history of attempted suicide
- Depression
- Hopelessness
- Patient demonstrates mood swings or acute psychotic behaviour
- Recent history of significant upset
- Currently under the influence of or withdrawing from drugs/alcohol

---

The initial management and treatment of deliberate self-harm (DSH)

Individuals who have committed an act of DSH are entitled to the same level of care, respect and privacy as all other patients. Caring for those who have intentionally injured themselves can lead to many personal feelings for practitioners; these can include frustration and anger, particularly when limited resources are available or if the patient has sabotaged a previous attempt to heal a wound. The wound itself or the act of self-harm are only the physical manifestation of this illness. In emergency care DSH is a disorder that initially requires a holistic approach, as purely addressing the physical side can prove futile. The initial rapport between the practitioner and the patient should comprise both, involving the patient in their care and empowering the patient to make decisions regarding their treatment and subsequent plan of care. A comprehensive assessment tool may expedite care and identify clinical urgency (RCP 2004). If relatives or friends accompany the patient, ask if they want to be consulted in private before commencing the consultation.

Definition and prevalence

DSH particularly among young people is a major public health issue, with estimations of one in 15 young people turning to DSH in times of crisis (National Inquiry into Self-harm among Young People 2006). There is much controversy over what constitutes mental illness, but most definitions contain similar characteristics, these include depression, anxiety, confusion and psychological trauma. These feelings, which can occur to anyone during particularly stressful periods of their life, occur to such an extent, or for a continual period of time, resulting in the affected individual finding it difficult to cope with everyday life. DSH is a symptom of a potentially serious underlying emotional or psychological trauma. Mental illness is very common, the DoH estimates that up to 5 per cent of emergency care presentations relate to a primary diagnosis of mental ill health (DoH 2004). The physical manifestation of this can be varied, although DSH and drug misuse are commonly implicated. A further 35 per cent of attendances relate to the effects of alcohol, including violent assaults, mental health emergencies and DSH (DoH 2004).

Deliberate self-harm (DSH)

DSH is a common reason for presentation to an ED. The physical manifestation of this type of presentation can range from minor cuts, scalding and scratches (in the case of Mr Johnson) through to life-threatening injuries such as stabbings, hangings and less focused self-mutilation such as poisoning and overdoses.

The Mental Health Act (MHA) (1983)

Occasionally patients will present acutely mentally ill and require detention under the Mental Health Act. There is strict guidance on the detention of patients with a multi-disciplinary approach being the key to success. Social work departments have a statutory responsibility regarding MH legislation; their role is pivotal as the implementer of MH law in most jurisdictions. Designated social workers can build close links between community services and the ED, which can prevent potential confusion and fragmentation of service delivery. Many local psychiatric services are community-based and are sited away from acute trusts. This has led to delays in specialist intervention and treatment, resulting in many cases of patients leaving the ED setting while awaiting specialist intervention. Current practice is aimed at preventing this, the DoH (2004) requirement that 90 per cent of patients attending with acute MH issues are seen and either admitted or discharged within four hours has instigated a dramatic change in clinical practice, directly improving the care of users. Despite this, the DoH (2004) identify that 10 per cent of patients remaining within an ED after four hours involve a mental health issue.

The MHA identifies periods when patients can be legally detained and treated due to mental illness, impairment or psychopathic behaviour. The detention must be based on necessity and in the interest of the patient or for the protection of others. Voluntary admission is preferable as it is not associated with the stigma and legal connotations of formal detention. The MHA does not relate to detaining patients for medical treatment (physical illness). If the treatment is considered to be in the patient's best interest, common law can be used to either keep a patient within the department or to ask police to trace and return a patient for essential treatment. Causes include acute confusional states discussed earlier and physical pathologies resulting in hypoxic changes. The head-injured patient demonstrating cerebral irritation, which manifests as aggressive and disrupted behaviour, demonstrates a common clinical example.

A patient attending with an acute MH illness will normally be detained under MHA Sections 2, 3 or 4. Section 2 is the most commonly used order and allows the patient to be detained for up to 28 days. While patients are awaiting the completion of legal papers, they should be detained under common law, although at no time should the practitioner risk their own safety. Hospital security should be used in conjunction with the police if necessary.

Most EDs are considered a place of safety and an acutely psychotic patient detained under Section 136 by the police may confront practitioners. This Section allows a police officer to detain and remove a patient to a 'place of safety' when in their opinion the patient is either a danger to themselves, or because of a potential mental illness a danger to the community at large. A patient should only be brought to the ED if that particular department has previously been designated a place of safety. This agreement should have been reached by the trust management in conjunction with representatives of the medical and nursing workforce and the police. This leads to a proficient service with pre-designated areas for care, and a structure to the event. The RCP (2004) have identified that many EDs are ill equipped for this purpose and therefore not a place of safety as it would not be in the patient's best interests to detain them there. If this is the case, the patient should be detained within a police station or transferred to a special area within a psychiatric unit (RCP 2004).

If the patient has been brought to the department for medical treatment, practitioners should ascertain the nature of the police involvement and under what circumstances they would remove the patient.

For in-depth discussion, the reader is referred to the RCP (2004).

It has been widely identified that there is currently a knowledge deficiency surrounding mental illness within EDs. Box 10.14 pinpoints some of the identified areas that can improve both the competence and confidence of practitioners and the care patients receive.

Box 10.14 Royal College of Psychiatrists' recommendations

- ED practitioners should have adequate knowledge of mental health (MH) issues to facilitate an initial assessment of an attendee with a primary mental health illness
- Staff training to include common MH issues and their initial management
- There should be close links between MH providers and EC staff
- Local policies should be available on common MH-related issues within the ED
- EDs should have a designated area for MH assessment, including adequate safety features
- Staff training should include safety issues
- A liaison group should facilitate networking between the two specialities to the benefit of all concerned, including the implementation of the recommendations of the RCP

(RCP 2004)

Conclusion

The assessment, treatment and overall management of emergency presentations related to an underpinning medical problem can be made extremely easy for emergency care staff by adopting a structured and evidence-based appoach. Current DoH policy is to increase the amount of national standards and care pathways enabling practitioners to gain competence and confidence in their clinical practice. Many EDs are one step ahead with senior staff taking the initiative and introducing local evidence-based standards to the benefit of patients and other members of the ED team. These multi-disciplinary pathways are easily audited and it is thereby easy to evaluate the care patients receive. New and junior members of the team are encouraged to familiarize themselves with local and national care pathways and guidelines as their use will expedite and rationalize frontline care delivery.

11 Paediatric emergencies

Jayne Gwyther

Introduction

Children account for approximately one-third of all patients seen in emergency departments (ED). Children account for between three and four million attendances per year. By their 5th birthday, 44 per cent of children will have attended an ED (Playfor 2001). Children attend with a wide spectrum of illness and injuries, from the trivial to the life-threatening (RCPCH 2002). They present a particular challenge to emergency practitioners, which calls for a prompt and accurate assessment.

Paediatric physiology differs from that of adults, enabling children to compensate in response to significant clinical illness. Conversely, however, this carries the risk that a severe problem may be overlooked or underestimated, when compensatory mechanisms fail in children, they often do so rapidly, catastrophically, and irreversibly (RCUK 2005).

This chapter aims to highlight the anatomical and physiological differences between children and adults; accurately recognize an unwell child using a rapid assessment approach; with reference to clinical scenarios, identify consent issues in caring for children; and, last, discuss child protection.

Box 11.1   Definition of ages in children
1   Infant: 0–1 year
2   Toddler: 1–3 years
3   Preschool: 3–5 years
4   School age: 6–12 years
5   Adolescent: >12 years
(RCUK 2005)

In this chapter when the term 'child' is used, this refers to all age ranges from birth to adolescence unless otherwise stated (Box 11.1).

Anatomical and physiological differences

Airway

The size of the airway is an important consideration as children have much smaller airways that can easily be obstructed; this is particularly relevant to infants, who are nasal breathers up until the age of six months. The anatomy of the airway changes with age, in all young children the epiglottis is horseshoe-shaped and projects posteriorly at 45 degrees, making intubation more difficult, for this reason during intubation straight blades are often chosen (RCUK 2005). In children, the cricoid ring is the narrowest part of the upper airway; within adults it is the larynx, as endotracheal tubes tend to lie at this level, uncuffed tubes are preferred in pre-pubertal children (RCUK 2005).

Care needs to be taken during intubation and suctioning as the paediatric airway has a delicate covering that is particularly prone to oedema if damaged. There is a high incidence of adenotonsillar hypertrophy in 3- to 8-year-olds that not only tends to cause obstruction but also causes difficulty when the nasal route is used to pass pharyngeal, gastric or tracheal tubes (RCUK 2005).

Breathing

Children have a higher metabolic rate and accompanying oxygen consumption that contributes to higher respiratory rates than in adults. Infants have ribs that lie more horizontally and they, therefore, depend predominately on diaphragmatic breathing and are more prone to muscle fatigue and consequently respiratory failure.

Circulation

Children have a comparatively smaller stroke volume (Chapter 2), and a higher cardiac output than adults; this is facilitated by higher heart rates (Table 11.1).

Table 11.1 Normal ranges of vital signs for age of child

	Age (years)			
	<1	2–5	5–12	>12
Pulse (bpm)	110–60	95–140	80–120	60–100
Respirations	30–40	25–30	20–5	15–20
Systolic BP (mmHg)	70–90	80–100	90–110	100–20

Source: RCUK (2005)

After the age of 2 the stroke volume increases with age, consequently heart rate falls. This is of particular significance in the shocked paediatric patient when compensatory mechanisms are failing. Children also have a lower systemic vascular resistance, evidenced by lower systolic blood pressure (Table 11.1).

The composition and distribution of body fluids differ with age: an infant has a greater content of extracellular fluid, with an increased exchange rate.

Other considerations

Children, and infants in particular, are at an increased risk of hypothermia due to both an immature temperature regulation system and their large surface area. Glycogen stores in the liver are limited and hypoglycaemia can be present in any paediatric patient who has been too ill to feed or subjected to high metabolic demands because of illness.

Recognition of the unwell child using a rapid assessment approach

The rapid assessment approach adopted for this chapter follows the same structure as previous chapters.

Airway

The patency of the airway must be assessed. Common causes of airway obstruction in children include displaced tongue, the presence of fluid or a foreign body, laryngeal oedema or trauma.

Noise can be an important factor in determining the cause and extent of obstruction: gurgling may indicate the presence of fluid such as blood or vomit in the main airways; snoring may suggest a partial occlusion of the pharynx by the tongue; an inspiratory stridor at the level of the larynx (voice box) may imply an upper airway obstruction. Complete airway obstruction in a child who is making respiratory effort is characterized by paradoxical chest and abdominal movements sometimes referred to as see-saw breathing (Chapter 9).

Work of breathing

Two rules exist when assessing the respiratory effort of a sick child:

1   Degree of recession *is* an indicator of severity of respiratory difficulty.
2   Volume of noise *is not* an indicator of severity of respiration difficulty.
(RCUK 2005)

Visual observation of the child can allow for an accurate assessment of the work of breathing and should include the following:

- Posture
- Evidence of altered behaviour
- Respiratory rate
- Colour
- Recession
- Respiratory noises.

Posture

Children in respiratory distress will tend to adopt a position that allows for maximum oxygenation. This can be referred to as the tripod or 'sniffing' position.

Evidence of altered behaviour

Children may present with a depressed conscious level or agitation. Caregivers will give an accurate account of the child's normal behaviour pattern: listen to them. Be concerned about any child in respiratory difficulty. This suggests they are fatigued and failing to compensate.

Respiratory rate and colour

Observe respiratory rate and rhythm. Central cyanosis (decreased oxygen saturation of haemoglobin in arterial blood) is best seen in buccal mucous membranes and lips. Peripheral cyanosis (slow blood circulation in fingers and toes) is best seen in nail beds (McCance and Huether 2002).

Recession

Intercostal and subcostal recession should be observed. Accessory muscle use occurs when the minute volume is high. This can be seen more easily in younger infants due to their compliant chest wall. The sick infant may display use of their sternomastoid (head bobbing) and abdominal-rectus muscles.

Respiratory noises

These can be good indicators of the cause. Inspiratory noise tends to be a sign of laryngeal or tracheal obstruction (upper airway), e.g., croup or epiglottitis. When confronted by a drooling child who is unable to swallow, a serious compromise of the airway should be expected. When suspecting epiglottitis or severe croup in a spontaneously breathing child, withhold all interventions. Do not attempt to examine the airway, use airway adjuncts or try to remove the child from their carer. Do not do anything that may increase distress. An expiratory noise (e.g., wheeze) indicates lower airway narrowing and will be more pronounced on expiration. An asthmatic child may present with a prolonged expiratory phase.

Indicative signs of severe respiratory distress especially in infants include:

1 Grunting: this is an attempt to generate a positive end-expiratory pressure (PEEP) to prevent airway collapse at the end of expiration.
2 Nasal flaring: this can be subtle and can be missed during the initial assessment.

Childhood asthma

> **Scenario 11.1**   Asthma in the child
>
> An 11-year-old girl attends the ED with a two-day exacerbation of asthma. The child's mother states the child has had an increase of wheezy episodes that have responded poorly to her inhalers.
>
> On arrival the child has marked respiratory distress with intercostal recession and a prolonged expiratory phase. Her respiratory rate is recorded as 42 breaths per minute, radial pulse is strong and fast at 170 bpm. She appears tired, breathless and unable to talk in sentences. She is warm to touch with a capillary refill of <2 seconds.

D *Data* (scientific facts): from the primary data the patient is currently portraying signs of acute severe asthma. This is confirmed by the presence of accessory muscle use with a prolonged expiratory phase and evidence of altered behaviour with the child appearing tired and too breathless to talk. The patient should be placed in an upright position and given high-flow oxygen via a face mask with a reservoir bag. Although strong, her pulse is fast and her respiratory rate elevated. An oxygen saturation probe should be used to ascertain the patient's oxygenation status and the oxygen saturation should be kept above 95 per cent. The patient's capillary refill time is currently <2 seconds indicating adequate circulation at this time.

E *Emotions* (intuition): when an unwell child attends the ED with acute respiratory distress, the possibility of the child's condition deteriorating cannot be overlooked. In this scenario the experienced assessor will sense the need for urgent action due to the level of respiratory distress and fatigue of the child. This will initiate further treatment within a high dependency area of the ED, thereby providing a suitable environment and adequate supervision.

A *Advantages*: children presenting with acute asthma are a common presentation to all emergency staff. This presentation should be taken seriously because without appropriate treatment and assessment, deterioration in condition will occur.

As with all acute severe episodes of asthma the nurse should commence high-flow oxygen and attach a pulse oximeter. Nebulized salbutamol (5mg) should be administered with oxygen at a flow rate of exceeding 6 litres a minute. Prednisolone 1.0 mg/kg (e.g., 30mg if child weighs 30kg) should be given if the child is able to tolerate oral medication. The child should be constantly observed and formally reassessed after 15–30 minutes; if there is no improvement a further salbutamol nebulizer should be given, and atrovent (250mcg) should be added (BTS and SIGN 2005).

D *Disadvantages* (**differential diagnoses**): the significance of the child being accurately assessed initially and receiving prompt, appropriate treatment cannot be over-emphasized. Remember some children with acute severe asthma will not appear distressed. If accurate assessment fails to take place, however, there is a risk of the child being placed in an area of the ED that does not allow for continual observation and appropriate treatment to occur.

Prevalence

The Asthma Audit 2001 showed that 1.4 million or 1 in 8 children in the UK today are receiving treatment for asthma. It is estimated that for every 100,000 patients in a primary care organization, there will be almost 4000 children diagnosed with asthma. Half of these will be visiting their GP at least once a year but more significantly, they will also accumulate 60 emergency hospital admissions each year (Asthma Audit 2002). Children will present in A&E units with varying degrees of severity, each requiring accurate assessment and appropriate treatment. It is worth noting that some children with acute severe asthma do not appear distressed. It can therefore be difficult to assess the severity of asthma because clinical signs correlate poorly with the severity of airway obstruction (RCUK 2005). The BTS and SIGN (2005) have set out clear guidance on classifying the severity of acute asthma in children and appropriate treatment (Table 11.2).

Asthma treatment in A&E

1   Initial treatment commences with the administration of high-flow oxygen via a face mask with a reservoir bag. It is worth noting that almost all sick children will benefit from high concentration oxygen therapy. There is no need to assess risk as in adults with chronic lung disease. Only a small group of infants with duct-dependent congenital heart disease need controlled oxygen therapy (Moulton and Yates 1999).

Table 11.2 Classification of acute asthma in children

Classification	Sign/symptom
Moderate asthma	• SaO2 >92%
	• No clinical features of severe or life-threatening asthma
	• Peak flow >50% best/predicted
Acute severe asthma	• Too breathless to feed or talk
	• Recession/use of accessory muscles
	• Respiratory rate >30/min (5 years)
	>50/min (2–5 years)
	• Pulse rate >120 beats/min (>5 years)
	>130 beats/min (2–5 years)
	• Peak flow <50% best/predicted
Life-threatening asthma	• Conscious level depressed/agitated
	• Exhaustion
	• Poor respiratory effort
	• SaO2 <92% in air/cyanosis
	• Silent chest
	• Peak flow <33% best/predicted
	• Hypotension

2   Attach a pulse oximeter and aim to keep SaO2 above 92 per cent.
3   Give a beta-2 agonist such as salbutamol:

  • For mild–moderate asthma give ten puffs via a spacer device. Inhalers should be sprayed into the spacer in individual puffs and inhaled by deep breathing generally 5–10 breaths per puff.
  • For severe–life-threatening asthma, give nebulized salbutamol.
  • 2.5 mg (<5 years) or 5 mg (>5 years) with oxygen at a flow rate of 4–6 l/min.

4   Give oral prednisolone 1.0 mg/kg or if vomiting IV hydrocortisone 4mg/kg.
5   If receiving nebulized salbutamol, combine with ipratropium bromide (atrovent) 250 mcg as per unit policy and drive with oxygen.
6   If not responding or the condition deteriorates, consider IV salbutamol. Monitor ECG and potassium levels for potential hypokalaemia.
7   If respiratory effort is poor or conscious level is depressed or SpO2 level falling, summon an anaesthetist and contact a PICU.

(RCUK 2005)

Cardiac arrest in childhood

Cardiac arrest is uncommon in children and usually occurs as a secondary complication of respiratory dysfunction or shock with prolonged hypoxia. Survival following a paediatric cardiac arrest is much lower than in adults. This is because the child will have sustained severe multiple system hypoxia before cardiac arrest develops. Early recognition of signs and symptoms of respiratory distress and shock are therefore essential so that arrest is prevented.

Facts about shock in children

1   Septic shock in meningococcal disease results from a loss of circulating plasma volume, maldistribution of intravascular volume, impaired myocardial function and impaired cellular metabolism. The child will present with signs and symptoms 'similar' to hypovolaemic shock.

2   Hypovolaemic shock is the most common type of shock in children. It is normally caused by dehydration and trauma but may also result from a redistribution of blood volume or increased capillary permeability following burns or sepsis (McCance and Huether 2002).

3   Hypovolaemia is a potentially reversible cause of cardiac arrest (RCUK 2005).

4   If hypovolaemia is suspected, infuse intravenous or intraosseous fluids rapidly. Use isotonic saline solutions, preferably 0.9 per cent normal saline. Avoid dextrose-based solutions as these will be redistributed rapidly away from the intravascular space and will cause hyponatraemia and hyperglycaemia which may worsen neurological outcome after cardiac arrest (RCUK 2005).

5   A human albumin solution of 4.5 per cent has been the main resuscitation fluid in meningococcal sepsis for several decades (Pollard et al. 1999).

6   Hypotension may not be observed in the child with shock unless intravascular loss is rapid or severe. This usually occurs with greater than 10 per cent dehydration in the infant or child or greater than 7 per cent in the adolescent.

7   A 20–5 per cent acute haemorrhage is usually required to produce hypotension in the child with trauma (McCance and Huether 2002). It is therefore important to look out for the earlier signs of shock before hypotension becomes evident.
    Hypotension is a late and pre-terminal sign of circulatory failure. Once a child's blood pressure has fallen, cardiac arrest is imminent.

8   The child in shock may have an altered capillary refill time (CRT). To accurately record an infant's CRT gently press on the forehead or sternum for 5 seconds rather than the peripheries where peripheral circulation can be delayed even in good health. CRT of less than 1.5–2 seconds is normal and may be observed in infants and children with minimal fluid deficit (less than 5 per cent dehydration). If the capillary refill time is 1.5–3 seconds in a warm room, a 5–10 per cent dehydration is likely to be present. A refill time over 3 seconds is associated with greater than 10 per cent dehydration. (McCance and Huether 2002).

9   Hypovolaemia can be classified into three stages:

- Compensated: During the compensated or early stage of shock vital organ function is maintained by instrinsic compensatory mechanisms.
- Decompensated: During the decompensated or late stage the efficiency of the cardiovascular system gradually diminishes.
- Irreversible: During the irreversible stage damage to vital organs is of such a magnitude that even despite therapeutic intervention, death occurs (McCance and Hueter 2002).

Signs and symptoms of shock

Compensated stage

1   Altered behaviour: carers may report an inability to settle the child with increased agitation, confusion or lethargy.
2   Pallor: a common early sign in shocked children.
3   Thirst.
4   Peripherally cool.
5   Unexplained tachycardia: a common early sign in 'shocked' children that *should not be ignored.*
6   Reduced urine output: urine output of less than 1ml/kg/hr in children and less than 2ml/kg/hr in infants indicates inadequate renal perfusion during shock.

Decompensated stage

1   Confusion.
2   Tachypnoea and tachycardia.
3   Moderate metabolic acidosis.
4   Oliguria.
5   Cool, pale extremities.
6   Decreased skin turgor.

7 Poor capillary refill.
8 A falling blood pressure.

(Wong et al. 2000)

Irreversible stage

1 Thready weak pulse.
2 Hypotension.
3 Periodic breathing or apnea.
4 Anuria.
5 Stupor or coma.

(Wong et al. 2000)

Meningococcal disease

Scenario 11.2 Meningococcal disease

A 2-year-old boy, accompanied by his mother, attends an ED with a 2-day history of coryza and loss of appetite. After an unsettled night, the child awoke this morning and appeared irritable and difficult to comfort. His mother recorded his temperature, which was 38 degrees centigrade. He was given paracetamol and placed back in his bed. Two hours later, when again appearing distressed, his mother noticed a rash on his leg. The GP was called who advised the mother to take the child to an ED immediately.

On arrival at the ED the child is drowsy with an elevated pulse of 185bpm and a respiratory rate of 40 per min. He is peripherally cool with a capillary refill of 4 seconds. A non-blanching rash is present on his lower right leg. He is pyrexial at 39.4 degrees centigrade. His blood pressure is stable at 90/40 mmhg.

D *Data* (scientific facts): from the primary data the child is displaying signs of meningococcal disease. This is recognizable due to the following signs: there is a non-blanching rash, which although may not always be present, remains one of the most common features; the child has an increased heart and respiratory rate and an alteration in mental status indicating the presence of shock; a prolonged capillary refill time and cool peripheries are also present. The child has a normal blood pressure which should *not* lead the ED practioner to believe the child is stable. Recognition of shock and prompt treatment are vital and may be life-saving in cases where meningococcal disease is suspected (Welch and Nadel 2003).

E *Emotions* (intuition): children with meningococcal disease can develop shock and/or raised intracranial pressure very rapidly (Welch and Nadel 2003). When an unwell child attends an ED with symptoms suggestive of this condition, it is imperative that the child is placed in a high dependency area of the department where prompt, appropriate treatment can commence. The paediatric team should be involved with the child's care at this stage. The anxiety of the child's care givers must be acknowledged. In this scenario the experienced assessor will be alert to the fact that the child is drowsy, has an elevated heart and respiratory rate and a non-blanching rash. These indicate that a rapid deterioration in this child's condition will be inevitable if treatment is not commenced immediately.

A *Advantages*: as with all children presenting with meningococcal disease, evaluation of airway, breathing and circulation should be made. Intravenous access should be secured immediately in order for the administration of antibiotics to occur. Intravenous antibiotics and fluid resuscitation should be commenced according to local protocol. In this scenario the child must be observed for signs of raised intracranial pressure and specialist paediatric advice should be sought.

D *Disadvantages* (**differential diagnoses**): children under the age of 3 years presenting with meningococcal disease may not always present with the more common signs of the illness (e.g., neck stiffness, photophobia, purpuric rash). Frequently nurses have to rely on intuition, observation skills and history from care givers in order to ascertain the initial condition of the child. In some cases due to the progression of the disease, some children require transfer to a regional paediatric intensive care unit where further specialist management can occur.

Prevalence

There are many conditions that precipitate shock in children. However, recognition of meningococcal disease – meningitis and septicaemia – appears to be one of the greatest challenges for A&E staff. It has become one of the most common infectious causes of death in children in the UK. Early diagnosis is crucial as the disease can progress so fast that within a few short hours of the initial symptoms appearing, a previously healthy child could be in intensive care fighting for their life (Meningitis Research Foundation 2002). This is worsened by the difficulty of detection in children under 3 years of age when the classic symptoms are rarely seen.

Box 11.2 Signs and symptoms of bacterial meningitis in infants and children

Infants: manifestations can be vague and non-specific:

1   Refuses feeds
2   Poor sucking ability
3   Vomiting or diarrhoea
4   Poor tone

5 Lack of movement
6 Poor cry
7 Full, tense bulging fontanelle – late sign
8 Convulsions
9 Drowsiness: altered behaviour, lack of eye contact with carer
10 Respiratory irregularities or apnoea

(Wong et al. 2000)

Children under 3 years of age:
1 Fever
2 Poor feeding
3 Marked irritability: altered behaviour, not easily soothed by carers
4 Restlessness
5 Convulsions
6 Purpuric rash
Neck stiffness, photophobia and positive Kernig's sign may be absent.

(Welch and Nadel 2003)

Older children of 4 years and over are more likely to have classic symptoms:
1 Headache
2 Vomiting
3 Pyrexia
4 Neck stiffness
5 Photophobia
6 Purpuric rash

Treatment of meningococcal disease in A&E

Immediate assessment

Children with meningococcal disease may develop shock and/or raised intra-cranial pressure (ICP) rapidly. For consistent management the responsible paediatric consultant should be involved in their care from the outset, and paediatric intensive care unit (PICU) advice should be sought early (Welch and Nadel 2003).

When the diagnosis is suspected, immediate evaluation of airway, breathing and circulation should be made, high-flow oxygen should be given via a face mask and resuscitation started as indicated. Intravenous access should be obtained as soon as possible (Welch and Nadel 2003), antibiotics (penicillin or a third-generation cephalosporin) should be given promptly either intramuscular or intravenous.

Treatment of shock

The goal of treating septic shock in meningococcal disease is to maintain tissue perfusion and oxygenation. The priority in achieving this is volume resuscitation to restore the intravascular compartment (Pollard et al. 1999).

Peripheral access in young children can be difficult and may be impossible in shock. If attempts at peripheral intravenous cannulation are unsuccessful after a few minutes, intraosseous access should be secured without delay. For fluid resuscitation, follow local protocol.

Treatment of raised intracranial pressure

Raised intracranial pressure (ICP) is a well recognized complication of meningitis. The signs include altered level of consciousness, bradycardia, hypertension or hypotension and altered respiratory pattern.

Transfer to intensive care

Initial resuscitation and stabilization may inevitably take place within the ED where the child first presents. Following this, some patients will require transfer to a regional paediatric intensive care unit. These will be the children who require intubation and ventilation for persistent shock. These children will require a secure airway, controlled mechanical ventilation, secure central venous and arterial access for ongoing cardiovascular support and monitoring (Welch and Nadel 2003).

Disability

A child's conscious level may be altered by disease, injury or intoxication, with head injury being one of the most common reasons for children to attend an ED (RCUK 2005). Children with a decreased conscious level are usually presented by parents who are very aware of the seriousness of the symptoms. They may also have noted other features such as headache, fever or exposure to poisoning which may aid diagnosis (RCUK 2005).

Because of variability in the definition of words describing the degree of coma, the Glasgow coma scale and the Children's coma scale have been developed as validated tools for the description of conscious states from all pathologies (RCUK 2005).

Assessing the child with a decreased conscious level

- What is the AVPU score? (Alert, response to Verbal stimuli, response to Pain, Unresponsive)
- What is their Glasgow coma scale score? In a previously well, unconscious child who is not in a post-ictal state, a score of <9 is suggestive of raised intracranial pressure (RCUK 2005)
- Is the child mobile? Do they run away? Or is there limited movement with poor muscle tone?
- Do they interact with carers or toys or are they uninterested or unresponsive, with altered behaviour?

- If they are crying or speaking, is this strong or weak?
- If crying, can they be consoled?
- Do they fix their gaze on responders or carers, or do they have a 'glazed' appearance?
- Is the child's behaviour normal for their developmental age?
- Do they have an abnormal posture? Decorticate or decerebrate posturing in a previously normal child should suggest raised intracranial pressure (RCUK 2005)
- Is the child fitting? This at times, especially in infants, can be subtle, therefore pay close attention during assessment – take time to observe all movements.
- Is the child stiff or floppy?

(Woollard and Jewkes 2004)

The fitting child

Scenario 11.3 Febrile convulsion

Archie, a 4-year-old boy is admitted ED following a 'fit' which lasted approximately 2 minutes, the fit resolved spontaneously. His mother states that for the past two days he has developed a temperature and chesty cough. Archie has no past medical history.

On arrival in the ED the child is spontaneously breathing and has an oxygen mask in situ. He has a pulse rate of 100 bpm and a respiratory rate of 48 per min. He is hot to touch and is producing large volumes of secretions.

D *Data* (scientific facts): the child on arrival is hot to touch, therefore possible bacterial infection must be ruled out at this stage and will require further investigation following the primary assessment. The mother is present and will be questioned regarding the nature of the convulsion prior to arrival in the ED. A specific point of interest will be the child's history of a cough and fever over the past two days.

E *Emotions* (intuition): in febrile convulsions death can occur through a number of causes including airway obstruction, severe hypoxia, aspiration of vomit, and effects of medication. The experienced ED practioner will be aware of the above complications and the set protocol of treatment that exists to treat febrile convulsions; because of this the child will be placed in a high dependency area of the ED where emergency management can occur. The longer the duration of the convulsion, the more difficult it is to terminate. It is usual practice to institute treatment when an episode has not ceased spontaneously in 5 minutes.

A *Advantages*: children arriving in the ED following a fit require an ABCDE assessment. In the scenario the child is spontaneously breathing and therefore following assessment of the airway for patency, high-flow oxygen should be continued. His blood glucose will be checked at this point. The child's breathing needs to be assessed for signs of difficulty, noting, in particular, signs of recession, rate and accessory muscle use. Vascular access should be secured for administration of medication and fluids. Anti-pyretics should be administered according to the weight-dependent dose to reduce the child's temperature and minimize the risk of further fits.

D *Disadvantages* (**differential diagnoses**): the child will require constant observation in order for possible complications to be recognized. The underlying cause of the convulsions will require investigation. Relevant to this scenario is a fever which suggests an infectious cause. If bacterial meningitis is suspected, the child must be commenced on antibiotic therapy according to local policy.

Exposure

External factors in relation to a child's presenting clinical signs must be taken into account in order to achieve an accurate assessment:

- Presence of a rash needs to be determined as part of the initial assessment. Carers are particularly vigilant regarding the existence of skin disorders and will often alert the practitioner. Diagnostic evaluation can often be made by gathering the history and observation of the distribution and characteristics of the presenting lesions (McCance and Huether 2002). Please note, with regard to meningococcal disease, up to 20 per cent of cases will have *no* rash or an atypical maculopapular rash (Welch and Nadel 2003).
- Presence of fever needs to be investigated. Many illnesses cause an elevation of body temperature and diagnosis needs to be finalized prior to discharging the child. *Every child with a fever and petechiae rash should be assumed to have meningococcal disease until proven otherwise* (Welch and Nadel 2003).
- Additional external factors may involve observation of swelling of the face and lips indicating possible anaphylaxis (RCUK 2005).

Consent and treatment

Children (that is patients under the age of 18) can be classified into three groups with respect to legal considerations regarding consent to treatment or its refusal:

- Minor over the age of 16
- Minor under the age of 16 who is 'Fraser competent'
- Minor under the age of 16 who is not 'Fraser competent'.

The doctrine of necessity may be applied, which may be particularly relevant to the A&E setting, if life-saving treatment is required for paediatric patients in any of these groups and consent cannot be obtained in a timely manner in the required way (Woollard and Jewkes 2004).

Minor over the age of 16

Children over the age of 16 should normally be treated as competent adults. Informed consent to treatment should be sought from the child. Adults with parental responsibility may not refuse treatment on behalf of the minor if the chid has consented to it. Adults with parental responsibility may, however, override the decision of a minor to refuse life-saving treatment, as may a court of law. If both a child and those with parental responsibility refuse life-saving treatment this can be retrospectively overruled by a court of law or, in an emergency, by health professionals (Woollard and Jewkes 2004).

A few notes about parental responsibility:

- The law relating to parental responsibility changed on 1 December 2003.
- In relation to children born before this date, both the child's legal parents have parental responsibility if they were married at the time of the child's conception or at sometime there after.
- If the parents have never married and the child was born before 1 December 2003, only the mother has parental responsibility. The father may acquire it in various ways, including entering into a parental responsibility agreement with the mother, or through a parental responsibility order made by the court.
- From 1 December 2003, unmarried fathers registered on the child's birth certificate will automatically get parental responsibility.
- If both parents have parental responsibility, neither loses it if they divorce, and responsibility endures if the child is in care or custody. It is lost if the child is adopted.
- A person other than the child's biological parents can acquire parental responsibility by being appointed as the child's guardian or by having a residence order made in his or her favour.
- A local authority acquires parental responsibility (shared with the parents) while the child is the subject of a care or supervision order.

Minor under the age of 16 who is 'Fraser competent'

In some circumstances, a child, under the age of 16, will be able to give consent without referral to their parents or carers if they are judged to be Fraser competent. The courts have stated that under-16s will be competent to give valid consent to a particular intervention if they have 'sufficient' understanding and intelligence to enable him or her to understand fully what is proposed. However, children under 16 should ideally be encouraged to involve their parent or carer unless to do so could put them at risk of harm (DFES 2005).

Minor under the age of 16 who is not 'Fraser competent'

When a minor under the age of 16 is deemed not to be Fraser competent, consent to treatment needs to be obtained from an adult with parental responsibility. If such an adult is not immediately available and treatment cannot be delayed, the legal doctrine of necessity may be invoked if treatment is necessary to save life, ensure improvement or prevent deterioration in health (Woollard and Jewkes 2004).

Safeguarding children in the ED

Everyone who comes into contact with children and families in their everyday work, including practitioners who do not have a specific role in relation to child protection, have a duty to safeguard and promote the welfare of children (DoH 2003). For ED staff the ability to recognize potential child abuse and respond appropriately to concerns cannot be overestimated.

What is child abuse?

A person may abuse or neglect a child by inflicting harm, or by failing to act to prevent harm. It is worth remembering that children and young people may be abused in a family, in an institutional or in a community setting (DOH 2003).

Four categories of child abuse exist:

1   *Physical abuse*
    This involves causing physical harm to a child, including the fabrication of symptoms, or deliberately causing ill health to a child.
2   *Neglect*
    This is the persistent failure to meet a child's basic physical and/or psychological needs, likely to result in the serious impairment of the child's health or development.

3 *Emotional abuse*

This is the persistent emotional ill-treatment of a child such as to cause severe persistent adverse effects on the child's emotional development. It may involve conveying to children that they are worthless or unloved, inadequate or valued only in so far as they meet the needs of another person.

4 *Sexual abuse*

This involves forcing or enticing a child or young person to take part in sexual activities, whether or not the child is aware of what is happening. The activities may involve physical contact, including penetrative or non-penetrative acts (DOH 2003).

Identifying potential abuse

Within child abuse certain aspects surrounding the event may be evident and should raise suspicion. The history may not be consistent with the injury and there may have been a delay in seeking medical help. The history may involve inconsistencies from care-givers who are vague, elusive, unconcerned or excessively distressed or aggressive. There may be recurrent injuries or injuries that are inconsistent with the child's stage of development (Lissauer and Clayden 2002).

Bruises are the commonest mode of presentation. Whereas bruises on the forehead and shins are common in toddlers learning to walk, they are exceptional in non-mobile babies. Bruises on the face, back and buttock are uncommon in genuine accidents. Some patterns of bruising are suggestive of particular injuries. Bruises from fingertips gripping with excessive force are mostly on the trunk, often either side of the spine, but may also be seen around the mouth from trying to stop a baby crying (Lissauer and Clayden 2002).

Burns and scalds are difficult to distinguish from those inflicted deliberately or accidental. Accidental hot water burns tend to be asymmetrical and spare the flexures and have splash marks. Scalds on the back are uncommon in accidents as are burns on the buttocks. The shape of the scald may be suggestive of the cause (e.g., a cigarette burn) (Lissauer and Clayden 2002).

Fractures can be categorized according to their likelihood of being caused by non-accidental injury. The most specific are fractures in infants, which require violent shaking or handling. It is the child's age, mobility and development that are the crucial features in distinguishing accidental from non-accidental injuries (Lissauer and Clayden 2002).

Only gross forms of neglect can be recognized in an ED. Some characteristics include short statue and underweight for age, poor skin condition (especially in the nappy area), dry sparse hair, lack of energy and failure to play, wasting and diarrhoea. Emotional abuse is even subtler than neglect

(Moulton and Yates 1999). It is imperative that these children are referred to specialist paediatric teams for further assessment and monitoring.

The sexual abuse of children can occur in all socio-economic, cultural and religious groups. Before the age of 16, at least one in ten girls and one in fifteen boys will have been sexually assaulted, the peak incidence of the first assault is around 8 years of age (Moulton and Yates 1999). Sexual abuse can be associated with acute perineal injury, sexually transmitted infections, sexually precocious behaviour, eating and sleep disorders, withdrawal and depression, running away from home and psychosomatic symptoms. A surprising number of patients who present with self-harm will later also give a history of sexual abuse (Moulton and Yates 1999).

What to do if you have concerns about a child

Most injuries presenting in ED follow genuine accidents and must, therefore, be differentiated from those which are inflicted deliberately.

- Discuss your concerns with senior colleagues and follow local policies and procedures.
- If you still have concerns following these discussions, refer the child to social services. Ideally seek to discuss with the child, as appropriate to their age and understanding, and with their parents and seek their agreement to making a referral to social services unless you consider such a discussion would place the child at risk of significant harm.
- When you make the referral, agree with the recipient of the referral what the child and parents will be told, by whom and when.
- If you make a referral by telephone, confirm it in writing within 48 hours. Social services should acknowledge your written referral within one working day of receiving it, so if you have not heard back within three working days, contact social services again.

(DOH 2003)

Conclusion

This chapter has discussed the many issues facing emergency practitioners who assess and care for children in an ED. Sick children require prompt accurate assessment if treatment is to be effective and appropriate. This chapter has aimed to highlight the differing needs of the unwell child and their carers and to support the emergency practitioner to recognize signs and symptoms of immediate concern.

List of figures, tables, boxes and scenarios

Figures

Tables

Boxes

Scenarios

References

Chapter 1

Alberti, G. (2004) *Transforming Emergency Care in England*. London: The Stationery Office.

Alfaro-LeFevre, R. (2004) *Critical Thinking and Clinical Judgement: A Practical Approach*. Philadelphia: Elsevier Science.

Andersson, A. K., Omberg, M. and Svedlund, M. (2006) Triage in the emergency department: a qualitative study of the factors which nurses consider when making decisions, *Nursing in Critical Care*, 11(3): 136–44.

Cioffi, J. (2000) Nurses' experiences of making decisions to call emergency assistance to their patients, *Journal of Advanced Nursing*, 32(1): 108–14.

DoH (Department of Health) (2000) *The NHS Plan: A Plan for Investment, a Plan for Reform*. London: The Stationery Office.

DoH (Department of Health) (2005) *A Guide to Emergency Medical and Surgical Admissions*. London: The Stationery Office.

Fonteyn, M. and Ritter, B. (2000) Clinical reasoning in nursing, in J. Higgs and M. Jones (eds) *Clinical Reasoning in the Health Professions*. Oxford: Butterworth Heinemann.

Franklin, C. and Matthew, J. (1994) Developing strategies to prevent in-hospital cardiac arrest: analysing responses of physicians and nurses in the hours before the event, *Critical Care Medicine*, 22: 244–7.

Geraci, E. B. and Geraci, T. P. (1994) An observational study of the emergency triage role in a managed care facility, *Journal of Emergency Nursing*, 20(3): 189–203.

Hodgetts, T. J., Kenward, G., Vlackoniklis, I. et al. (2002) Incidence, location and reasons for avoidable in-hospital cardiac arrest in a district general hospital, *Resuscitation*, 54(2): 115–23.

McCaig, L. F. and Burt, C. W. (1999) National hospital ambulatory medical survey: emergency department summary, *Advanced Data 2001*, 320: 1–36.

NMC (Nursing and Midwifery Council) (2004) *Code of Professional Conduct: Standards for Conduct, Performance and Ethics*. London: NMC.

RCUK (Resuscitation Council UK) (2006) *Advanced Life Support Course Provider Manual*, 6th edn. London: Resuscitation Council UK.

Tippins, E. (2005) How emergency department nurses identify and respond to critical illness, *Emergency Nurse*, 13(3): 24–33.

Travers, D. (1999) Triage: how long does it take? How long should it take? *Journal of Emergency Nursing*, 25: 238–41.

Chapter 2

American College of Surgeons (2004) *Advance Trauma Life Support for Doctors*, 7th edn. Chicago: American College of Surgeons.

Annane, D., Bellissant, E. and Edouard, E. et al. (2004) Corticosteriods for severe sepsis and septic shock: a systematic review and meta-analysis, *British Medical Journal*, 239: 480.

Clancy, J. and McVicar, A.J. (2002) *Physiology and Anatomy: A Homeostatic Approach*, 2nd edn. London: Arnold.

Evans, C. and Tippins, E. (2005) Emergency treatment of anaphylaxis, *Accident and Emergency Nursing*, 13(4): 232–7.

Guidet, B., Aegerter, P., Gauzit, R., Meshaka, P. and Dreyfuss, D. (2005) Incidence and impact of organ dysfunction associated with sepsis, *Chest*, 127: 942–51.

Mallett, J. and Bailey, C. (1996) *The Royal Marsden NHS Trust Manual of Clinical Nursing Procedures*, 4th edn. Oxford: Blackwell Science.

Marieb, E.N. (1992) *Human Anatomy and Physiology*, 2nd edn. New York: Benjamin/ Cummings Publishing Company Inc.

Pepe, P. (2003) Shock in polytrauma, *British Medical Journal*, 327: 1119–20.

RCUK (Resuscitation Council UK) (2006) *Advanced Life Support*, 5th edn. London: RCUK

Tippins, E. (2005) How emergency department nurses identify and respond to critical illness, *Emergency Nurse*, June, 3(3): 24–33.

Vernooy, K., Verbeek, X., Peschar, M. et al. (2005) Left bundle branch block induces ventricular remodelling and functional septal hypoperfusion, *European Heart Journal*, 26: 91–8.

Chapter 3

AHA (American Heart Association) (2006) Heart disease and stroke statistics 2006 update: a report from the American Heart Association Statistics Committee and Stroke Statistics Subcommittee, *Circulation*, 113: 85–151.

BHF (British Heart Foundation) (2005) *Coronary Heart Disease Statistics*. Oxford: British Heart Foundation Health Promotion Research Group Department of Public Health, University of Oxford.

Bilal Iqbal, M., Taneja, A.K. and Lip, G.Y.H. (2005) Recent developments in atrial fibrillation, *British Medical Journal*, 330: 238–43.

DoH (Department of Health) (2000) *National Service Framework for Coronary Heart Disease*. London: The Stationery Office.

DoH (Department of Health) (2001) *Reforming Emergency Care*. London: The Stationery Office.

DoH (Department of Health) (2004) *Winning the War on Heart Disease*. London: The Stationery Office.

ESC (European Society of Cardiology) (2005) Guidelines for percutaneous coronary intervention, *European Heart Journal*, 26: 804–47.

Ezekowitz, M.D. (1999) Atrial fibrillation: the epidemic of the new millennium, *Annual of Internal Medicine*, 131: 537–8.

Ghuran, A., Uren, N. and Nolan, J. (2003) *Emergency Cardiology: An Evidenced-Based Guide to Acute Cardiac Problems*. London: Arnold.

Houghton, A. and Gray, D. (2003) *Making Sense of the ECG: A Hands On Guide*, 2nd edn. London: Arnold.

Majeed, A., Moser, K. and Carroll, K. (2001) Trends in the prevalence and management of atrial fibrillation in general practice in England and Wales, 1994–1998: analysis of data from the general practice research database, *Heart*, 86: 284–8.

MINAP (Myocardial Infarction National Audit Project) (2004) *How Hospitals Manage Heart Attacks: Third Public Report of the Myocardial Infarction National Audit Project*. London: Clinical Effectiveness and Evaluation Unit, Royal College of Physicians.

NICE (National Institute for Clinical Excellence) (2004) *Clopidogrel in the Treatment of Non-ST-Segment-Elevation Acute Coronary Syndrome*. London: NICE.

RCUK (Resuscitation Council UK) (2006) *Advanced Life Support*, 5th edn. London: RCUK.

Saladin, K. (2005) *Human Anatomy*, International Edition. New York: McGraw-Hill.

Stewart, S., Murphy, N., Walker, A., McGuire, A. and McMurray, J.J.V. (2004) Cost of an emerging epidemic: an economic analysis of atrial fibrillation in the UK, *Heart*, 90: 286–92.

The Task Force for Percutaneous Coronary Interventions of the European Society of Cardiology (2005) Guidelines for percutaneous coronary intervention, *European Heart Journal*, 26: 804–47.

Chapter 4

Begg, J.D. (2005) *Accident and Emergency X-rays Made Easy*. London: Churchill Livingstone

British Medical Journal (2003) 326: 418.

Cooper, D., Moran, C., Everett, M., Lonstaff, P. and Riddle, W.H. (1997) Treatment methods for grade 1 ankle injuries, *Emergency Nurse*, 5(4): 21–3.

Cross, S. and Rimmer, M. (2002) *Nurse Practitioner: Manual of Clinical Skills*. Edinburgh: Balliere Tindall.

DoH (Department of Health) (2001) *Reforming Emergency Care*. London: The Stationery Office.

DoH (Department of Health) (2006) *Modernising Emergency Care Minor Illness and Injury* at. www.dh.gov.uk/PolicyAndGuidance/OrganisationPolicy/ EmergencyCare/ModernisingEmergencyCare/ModernisingEmergencyCare Article/fs/en?CONTENT_ID=4063813&chk=cB44Sc (accessed 13 June 2006).

Purcell, D. (2003) *Minor Injuries: A Clinical Guide for Nurses*. Edinburgh: Churchill Livingstone.

Saladin, K. (2005) *Human Anatomy*, International edn. New York: McGraw-Hill.

Stiell, I., Greenburg, G., McKnight, R., et al. (1992) A study to develop clinical decision rules for the use of radiography in acute ankle injuries, *Annals of Emergency Medicine*, 21(4): 55–61.

Stiell, I. et al. (1997) Implementation of the Ottawa Knee rules for the use of radiography in acute knee injuries, *Journal of American Medical Association*, 278(23): 2075–9.

Chapter 5

American College of Surgeons (2004) *Advance Trauma Life Support for Doctors*, 7th edn. Chicago: American College of Surgeons.

Dickinson, M. (2004) Understanding the mechanism of injury and kinetic forces involved in traumatic injuries, *Emergency Nurse*, 12(6): 30–4.

Harris, M. and Sethi R (2006) The initial assessment and management of the multiple-trauma patient with an associated spine injury, *Spine*, 31(Supplement 11): S9–S15.

Hawley, J., Dreher, M. and Vasso, M. (2003) Under pressure: treating cardiac tamponade, *Nursing Management*, 34(2): 44D, 44F, 44H.

Jansen, J. and Logie, J. (2005) Diagnostic peritoneal lavage: an obituary, *British Journal of Surgery*, 92(5): 517–18.

Kauver, D. and Wade, C. (2005) The epidemiology and modern management of traumatic hemorrhage: US and international perspectives, *Critical Care*. 9(Supplement 5): S1–S9.

Krausz, M. (2006) Initial resuscitation of hemorrhagic shock, *World Journal of Emergency Surgery*, 10: 1186/1749–7922–1–14.

Kwann, I., Bunn, F. and Roberts, I. (2003) *Timing and Volume of Fluid Administration for Patients with Bleeding (Review)* (On behalf of the WHO Pre-Hospital Trauma Care Steering Committee: The Cochrane Collaboration). London: John Wiley & Sons, Ltd

Laws, D., Neville, E. and Duffy, J. (2003) BTS guidelines for the insertion of a chest drain, *Thorax*, 58(Supplement II): II53–II59.

Leigh-Smith, S. and Harris, T. (2005) Tension pneumothorax: time for a re-think? *Emergency Medicine Journal*, 22: 8–16.

Ollerton, J., Sugrue, M., Balogh, Z., et al. (2006) Prospective study to evaluate the influence of FAST on trauma patient management, *Trauma*, 60(4): 785–91.

Royal College of Surgeons of England (1988) *The Management of Patients with Major Injuries*. London: Royal College of Surgeons.

WHO (World Health Organization) (2004) *Guidelines for Essential Trauma Care*. Geneva: WHO.

Chapter 6

Baker, P. (2006) *Obstetrics by Ten Teachers*, 18th edn. London: Hodder Arnold.

Benzoni, T. (2006) *Pregnancy, Delivery*: Emedicine. Available at: http://www.emedicine.com/emerg/topic477.htm

Chamberlain, G. and Steer, P. (1999) ABC of labour care: obstetric emergencies, *British Medical Journal*, 318: 1342–5.

Cox, C., Grady, K. and Hinshaw, K. (2003) *Managing Gynaecological Emergencies*. Oxford: BIOS Scientific Publishers Ltd.

Ectopic Pregnancy Trust (2004) *For Women Who Have Had or Suspect They May Have an Ectopic*. Available at: http://www.ectopic.org

Gilling-Smith, C., Toozs-Hobson, P., Potts, D.J., Touquet, R., and Beard, R.W. (1994) Management of bleeding in early pregnancy in accident and emergency departments, *British Medical Journal*, 309(6954): 574–5.

Govan, A. and Garrey, M. (eds) (1985) *Gynaecology Illustrated*, 3rd edn. Edinburgh: Churchill Livingstone.

Gould, D. (2004) Benign ovarian neoplasms, *Nursing Standard*, 18(17): 45–52, 54–55.

Lewis, G. and Drife, J. (eds) (2002) *Why Mothers Die 2000–20002. Report of the Sixth Confidential Enquiry into Maternal & Child Health (CEMACH): Improving the Health of Mothers, Babies and Children*. London: RCOG.

Lewis, T. and Chamberlain, G. (1989) *Gynaecology by Ten Teachers*. London: Edward Arnold.

Miscarriage Association (2005) *The Miscarriage Association: About Pregnancy Loss*. Available at: http://www.miscarriageassociation.org.uk/

Oláh, K. (2003) *Atlas of Gynaecology*. London: Royal College of Obstetricians and Gynaecologists.

Pitkin, J., Peattie, A. and Magowan, B. (2003) *Obstetrics & Gynaecology: An Illustrated Colour Text*. London: Churchill Livingstone.

RCOG (2002) *Setting Standards to Improve Women's Health*. Available at: http://www.rcog.org.uk/

RCUK (Resuscitation Council UK) (2006) *Advanced Life Support*, 5th edn. London: RCUK.

Rosevear, S. (2002) *Handbook of Gynaecology Management*. Cornwall: Blackwell Science.

Smeltzer, S.C. and Bare, B.G. (2004) *Brunner and Suddarth's Textbook of Medical–Surgical Nursing*. Philadelphia: Lippincott Williams & Wilkins.

Sorinola, O. and Cox, C. (2002) Accidents to ovarian cysts, *The Obstetrician & Gynaecologist*, 1(1). 10–13.
Steer, P. and Flint, C. (1999) ABC of labour care: physiology and management of normal labour, *British Medical Journal*, 318: 793–6.
Weckstein, L. N., Boucher, A. R., Tucker, H. (1995) Accurate diagnosis of early ectopic pregnancy, *Obstetrics & Gynaecology*, 65: 393–7.

Chapter 7

Albarran, J. (2002) The language of chest pain, *Nursing Times*, 98(4): 38–40.
Anagnostou, T. and Tolley, D. (2004) Management of ureteric stones, *European Urology*, 45: 714–21.
Birchley, D. (2006) Patients with clinical acute appendicitis should have pre-operative full blood count and C-reactive protein assays, *Annals of the Royal College of Surgeons of England*, 88(1): 27–32.
Cardall, T., Glaser, J. and Gus, D.A. (2004) Clinical value of the total white blood cell count and temperature in the evaluation of patients with suspected appendicitis, *Academic Emergency Medicine*, 11: 1021–7.
Epstein, O., Perkins, G.D., Cookson, J. and de Bono, D.P. (2003) *Clinical Examination*, 3rd edn. Edinburgh: Mosby.
Fagan, S.P., Awad, S.S., Rahwan, K., et al. (2003) Prognostic factors for the development of gangrenous cholecystitis. *The American Journal of Surgery*, 186: 481–5.
Habib, N. and Canelo, R. (2005) Liver and biliary tree, in M.J. Henry and J.N. Thompson (eds) *Clinical Surgery*, 2nd edn. Edinburgh: Elsevier Saunders.
Liang, MK. (2005) The art and science of diagnosing acute appendicitis, *Southern Medical Journal*, 98(12): 1159–60.
Lin, C., Chen, J., Tiu, C. et al. (2005) Can ruptured appendicitis be detected preoperatively in the ED? *American Journal of Emergency Medicine*, 23: 60–6.
Marieb, E.N. and Hoehn, K. (2007) *Human Anatomy and Physiology*, 7th edn. San Francisco: Pearson Benjamin Cummings.
McEntee, G.P. (1999) Small bowel obstruction, in J. Monson, G. Duthie, and K. O'Malley (eds) *Surgical Emergencies*. Oxford: Blackwell Science.
McHale, P.M. and LoVecchio, F. (2001) Narcotic analgesia in the acute abdomen: a review of prospective trials, *European Journal of Emergency Medicine*, 8(2): 131–6.
Ohki, T. and Veith, F.J. (2004) Endovascular repair of ruptured AAAs, *Endovascular Today*, January, pp. 47–51.
O'Kelly, T.J. and Krukowski, Z.H. (1999) The acute abdomen and laparotomy, in J. Monson, G. Duthie and K. O'Malley (eds) *Surgical Emergencies*. Oxford: Blackwell Science.
Parker, P. (2004) Acute pancreatitis, *Emergency Nurse*, 11(10): 28–35.
Pasero, C. (2003) Pain in the emergency department: withholding pain medication is not justified, *American Journal of Nursing*, 103(7): 73–4.

Ripolles, T., Agramunt, M., Errando, J. et al. (2004) Suspected ureteral colic: plain film and sonography vs unenhanced helical CT – a prospective study in 66 patients, *European Radiology*, 14(1): 129–36.

Shikata, S., Noguchi, Y. and Fukui, T. (2005) Early versus delayed cholecystectomy for acute cholecystitis: a meta-analysis of randomized controlled trials, *Surgery Today*, 35(7): 553–60.

Shokeir, A.A. (2002) Renal colic: new concepts related to pathophysiology, diagnosis and treatment, *Current Opinion in Urology*, 12(4): 263–9.

Teichman, J.M.H. (2004) Acute renal colic from ureteral calculus, *The New England Journal of Medicine*, 350(7): 684–93.

Thompson, J.N. (2005) Small-bowel disease and intestinal obstruction, in M.J. Henry and J.N. Thompson (eds) *Clinical Surgery*, 2nd edn. Edinburgh: Elsevier Saunders.

Tjandra, J.J. (2006) The appendix and Meckel's diverticulum, in J.J. Tjandra, G.J.A. Clunie, A.H. Kaye and J.A. Smith (eds) *Textbook of Surgery*, 3rd edn. Oxford: Blackwell Publishing.

Worster, A. and Richards, C. (2005) Fluids and diuretics for acute ureteric colic, *The Cochrane Database of Systematic Reviews*, (3): CD004926.

Chapter 8

American College of Surgeons (2004) *Advance Trauma Life Support for Doctors*, 7th edn. Chicago: American College of Surgeons.

Langlois, J.A., Rutland-Brown, W. and Thomas, K.E. (2004) *Traumatic Brain Injury in the United States: Emergency Department Visits, Hospitalisations, and Deaths.* Atlanta (GA): Centers for Disease Control and Prevention, National Center for Injury Prevention and Control.

McQuillan, K., Von Rueden, K., Hartsock, R., Flynn, M. and Whalen, E. (2002) *Trauma Nursing: From Resuscitation Through Rehabilitation*, 3rd edn. Philadelphia: W. B. Saunders Company.

NICE (National Institute for Clinical Excellence) (2003). *Head Injury Triage, Assessment, Investigation and Early Management of Head Injury in Infants, Children and Adults: Clinical Guideline 4.* London: NICE.

Saladin, K. (2005) *Human Anatomy*, International edn. New York: McGraw-Hill.

Shire, D., Poutler, J. and Lewis, R. (2004) *Hole's Human Anatomy and Physiology*, 10th edn. New York: McGraw-Hill.

Sultan, H.Y., Boyle, A., Pereira, M., Antoun, N. and Maimaris, C. (2004) Application of the Canadian CT head rules in managing minor head injuries in a UK emergency department: implications for the implementation of the NICE guidelines, *Emergency Medical Journal*, 21: 420–5.

Teasdale, G. and Jennett, B. (1974) Assessment of coma and impaired consciousness: a practical scale, *Lancet*, 2: 81–4.

Chapter 9

American College of Surgeons (2004) *Advance Trauma Life Support for Doctors*, 7th edn. Chicago: American College of Surgeons.

BTS (British Thoracic Society) (2004) *BTS Guidelines for the Management of Community Acquired Pneumonia in Adults*. London: BTS.

BTS (British Thoracic Society) and SIGN (Scottish Intercollegiate Guidelines Network) (2005) *British Guidelines on the Management of Asthma: A National Clinical Guideline*, revised edn. London: BTS and SIGN.

Cates, C. (2001) Extracts from *Clinical Evidence*: chronic asthma, *British Medical Journal*, 323: 976–9.

Currie, G.P., Devereux, G.S., Lee, D.K.C. and Ayres, J.G. (2005) Recent developments in asthma management, *British Medical Journal*, 330: 585–9.

Global Initiative for Asthma (GINA) (2004) *Global Strategy for Asthma Management and Prevention*, NIH Publication No. 02–3659.

Johnson, J.E., Gavin, D.J. and Adams-Dramiga, S. (2002) Effects of training with heliox and non-invasive positive pressure ventilation on exercise ability in patients with severe COPD, *Chest*, 122: 464–72.

Kleinschmidt, P. (2005) *Chronic Obstructive Pulmonary Disease and Emphysema: Emedicine*. Available at: http://www.emedicine.com/emerg/topic99.htm (accessed 12 May 2006).

NICE (National Institute for Clinical Excellence) (2004) *NICE Guideline to Improve Care of Patients with Chronic Obstructive Pulmonary Disease*. London: NICE.

Pellerano, M.E. (2005) Fast facts: respiratory tract infection, *Chest*, 127: 693–4.

Poponick, J., Renston, J.P., Bennett, R.P. and Emerman, C.L. (1999) Use of a ventilatory support system (BIPAP) for acute respiratory failure in the emergency department, *Chest*, 116: 166–71.

RCUK (Resuscitation Council UK) (2006) *Advanced Life Support*, 5th edn. London: RCUK.

Shire, D., Poutler, J. and Lewis, R. (2004) *Hole's Human Anatomy and Physiology*, 10th edn. New York: McGraw-Hill.

Vanpee, D., Khawand, C., Rousseau, L. et al. (2002) Effects of nasal pressure support on ventilation and inspiratory work in normocapnic and hypercapnic patients with stable COPD, *Chest*, 122: 75–83.

Chapter 10

ADA (American Diabetes Association) (2005) Standards of medical care in diabetes, *Diabetes Care*, 28 (Supplement I).

AHA (American Heart Association) (2006) Heart disease and stroke statistics: a report from the American Heart Association Statistics Committee and Stroke Statistics Subcommittee, *Circulation*, 113: 85–151.

Anionwu, E. and Atkin, K. (2001) *The Politics of Sickle Cell and Thalassaemia*. Buckingham: Open University Press.

ASA (American Stroke Association) (2006) Guidelines for prevention of stroke in patients with ischemic stroke or transient ischemic attack, *Stroke*, 37(2): 577–617.

Australasian College for Emergency Medicine (2005) *Guidelines on the Implementation of the Australasian Triage Scale in Emergency Departments*, revised edn. Melbourne: Australasian College for Emergency Medicine.

BHF (British Heart Foundation) (2006) *Coronary Heart Disease Statistics*. Oxford: British Heart Foundation Health Promotion Research Group, Department of Public Health, University of Oxford.

BSG (British Society of Gastroenterology) (2006) *Care of Patients with Gastrointestinal Disorders in the United Kingdom: A Strategy for the Future*. London: BSG.

BSGEC (British Society of Gastroenterology Endoscopy Committee) (2002) *GUT*, 51(supplement IV): IV1–IV6.

BTS (British Thoracic Society Standards of Care Committee, Pulmonary Embolism Guideline Development Group) (2003) British Thoracic Society guidelines for the management of suspected acute pulmonary embolism, *Thorax*, 58: 470–84.

Clancy, J. and McVicar, A.J. (2002) *Physiology and Anatomy: A Homeostatic Approach*, 2nd edn. London: Arnold.

Claster, S. and Vichinsky, E.P. (2003) Managing sickle cell disease, *British Medical Journal*, 327: 1151–5.

Dallal, H. and Palmer, K.R. (2001) ABC of the upper gastrointestinal tract: upper gastrointestinal haemorrhage, *British Medical Journal*, 323: 1115–77.

DoH (Department of Health) (2001a) *National Service Framework for Older People*. London: The Stationery Office.

DoH (Department of Health) (2001b) *National Service Framework for Diabetes: Standards*. London: The Stationery Office.

DoH (Department of Health) (2003) *National Service Framework for Diabetes: Delivery Strategy*. London: The Stationery Office.

DoH (Department of Health) (2004) *Improving the Management of Patients with Mental Ill Health in Emergency Care Settings*. London: The Stationery Office.

DoH (Department of Health) (2005) *Improving Diabetes Services: The NSF Two Years On*. London: The Stationery Office.

DoH (Department of Health) (2006) *Turning the Corner: Improving Diabetes Care*. London: The Stationery Office.

English, P. and Williams, G. (2004) Hyperglycaemia crises and lactic acidosis in diabetes mellitus, *Postgraduate Medical Journal*, 80: 253–61.

Gladwin, M.T., Schechter, A.N., Shelhamer, J.H. and Ognibene, F.P. (1999) The acute chest syndrome in sickle cell disease: possible role of nitric oxide in its pathophysiology and treatment, *American Journal of Critical Care Medicine*, 159: 1368–76

Gow, P.J. and Chapman, R.W. (2001) Modern management of oesophageal varices, *Postgraduate Medical Journal*, 77: 75–81.

Lilienfeld, D.E. (2000) Decreasing mortality from pulmonary embolism in the United States, 1979–1996, *International Journal of Epidemiology*, 29: 465–9.

Munro, P., Smith, R. and Parke, R. (2002) Effect of patients' age on management of acute intracranial haematoma: prospective national study, *British Medical Journal*, 325: 1001.

NAO (National Audit Office) (2005) *Reducing Brain Damage: Faster Access to Better Stroke Care*. London: The Stationery Office.

National Inquiry into Self-harm Among Young People (2006) *Truth Hurts: Fact or Fiction?* London: Camelot Foundation and the Mental Health Foundation.

NICE (National Institute for Clinical Excellence) (2004a) *Dyspepsia: Management of Dyspepsia in Adults in Primary Care*. London: NICE.

NICE (National Institute for Clinical Excellence) (2004b) *Self-harm: The Short-term Physical and Psychological Management and Secondary Prevention of Self-harm in Primary and Secondary Care*. London: National Collaborating Centre for Mental Health, NICE.

NIH (National Institute of Health) and NHLBI (National Heart, Lung, and Blood Institute) (2002) *The Management of Sickle Cell Disease*, 4th edn. New York: NIH.

ONS (Office of National Statistics) (2006) Heart disease leading cause of death in England and Wales, *Health Statistics Quarterly*, Summer.

Ramrakha, P. and Moore, K. (2004) *Oxford Handbook of Acute Medicine*, 2nd edn. Oxford: Oxford University Press.

RCP (Royal College of Physicians) (2004) *National Clinical Guidelines for Stroke*, 2nd edn. London: Intercollegiate Stroke Working Party, RCP.

RCP (Royal College of Psychiatrists) (2004) *Psychiatric Services to Accident and Emergency Departments*, Council Report CR118. London: British Association for Accident and Emergency Medicine, RCP.

Saladin, K. (2005) *Human Anatomy*, International edn. New York: McGraw-Hill.

Slater, D. and Johns, J. (2003) *Middle Cerebral Artery Stroke: Emedicine*. Available at: http://www.emedicine.com/pmr/topic77.htm (accessed 12 April 2006).

Stewart, J. Dundas, R. Howard, R.S. Rudd, A.G. and Wolfe, C.D.A. (1999) Ethnic differences in incidence of stroke: prospective study with stroke register, *British Medical Journal*, 318: 967–71.

WHO (World Health Organization) (1996) *WHO Guidelines: Cancer Pain Relief*, 2nd edn. Geneva: World Health Organization.

WHO (World Health Organization) (1999) *Definition, Diagnosis and Classification of Diabetes Mellitus and its Complications: Report of a WHO Consultation, Part 1*. Geneva: Department of Noncommunicable Disease Surveillance, WHO.

Chapter 11

Advanced Trauma Life Support for Doctors (2004) *Student Course Manual*, 7th edn. New York: American College of Surgeons.

Asthma Audit (2002) *Children with Asthma*. Available at: www.asthma.org.uk/about/factsheet38.php (accessed 15 February 2006).

Bashir, H.E., Laundy, M. and Booy, R. (2003) Diagnosis and treatment of bacterial meningitis, *Archives of Disease in Childhood*, 88: 615–20.

BTS (British Thoracic Society) and SIGN (Scottish Intercollegiate Guidelines Network) (2005) *British Guidelines on the Management of Asthma: A National Clinical Guideline*. Revised edn. London: BTS and SIGN.

DfES (Department of Education and Skills) (2005) *Training for Users of the Common Assessment Framework (CAF): Trainer Notes for Section 3*, Pilot version, May. London: DfES.

DoH (Department of Health) (2003) *What to Do if You're Worried a Child is Being Abused*. London: The Stationery Office.

Emergency Paediatric Care (undated) *The Practical Approach*, CD-ROM. Oxford: Blackwell Publishing.

Gill, D. and O'Brien, N. (2003) *Paediatric Clinical Examination Made Easy*, 4th edn. Edinburgh: Churchill Livingstone.

Hazinski, M.F. (1992) *Nursing Care of the Critically Ill Child*, 2nd edn. New York: Mosby.

Kurfis Stephens, B., Barkey, M. and Hall, H. (1999) Techniques to comfort children during stressful procedures, *Accident and Emergency Nursing*, 7: 226–36

Lissauer,T. and Clayden, G (2002) *Illustrated Text Book of Paediatrics*, 2nd edn. London: Mosby.

McCance, K. and Huether, S. (2002) *Pathophysiology: The Biologic Basis for Disease in Adults and Children*, 4th edn. London: Mosby.

Meningitis Research Foundation (2002) Available at: www.meningitis.org/news/newsitem (accessed 7 February 2006).

Moulton, C. and Yates, D. (1999) *Lecture Notes on Emergency Medicine*, 2nd edn. London: Blackwell.

Playfor, S. (2001) Accident and Emergency Services for Children within Trent Region, *Emergency Medicine Journal*, 18: 164–6.

Pollard, A.J., Britto, J., Nadel, S. et al. (1999) Emergency management of meningococcal disease, *Archives of Disease in Childhood*, 80: 290–6.

RCPCH (Royal College of Paediatrics and Child Health) (2002) *Children's Attendance at a Minor Injury/Illness Service*. London: RCPCH.

RCUK (Resuscitation Council UK) (2005) *Paediatric Advanced Life Support*. London: Resuscitation Guidelines.

Welch, S.B. and Nadel, S. (2003) Treatment of meningococcal infection, *Archives of Disease in Childhood*, 88: 608–14.

Wong, D.L., Hockenberry, M.J., Wilson, D. and Winkelstein, M.L. (2000) *Wong's Essentials of Pediatric Nursing*, 6th edn. London: MOSBY.

Woollard, M. and Jewkes, F. (2004) Assessment and identification of paediatric primary survey positive patients, *Emergency Medical Journal*, 21: 511–17.

Index

Related books from Open University Press

Purchase from www.openup.co.uk or order through your local bookseller

THE USE OF COUNSELLING SKILLS IN THE EMERGENCY SERVICES

Angela Hetherington

This book examines the use of counselling skills in the unique working environment of the emergency services. It looks at the stress and trauma of emergency service work, and draws extensively on the first hand experiences of personnel. The text considers how counselling skills can be employed effectively by emergency service professionals to enable them to fulfil their primary roles. In addition the book discusses the trained use of counselling skills within a formal peer support program and by management.

A major theme throughout the book is the psychological impact of traumatic incidents both on the victims and those involved in their rescue and recovery. This text considers the specific use of counselling skills in response to traumatic incidents, from a professional, ethical and legal perspective. It will be of use to Fire, Police, Accident and Emergency, Ambulance and Security Services and to voluntary emergency services such as The British Red Cross.

Contents
Preface – Counselling skills in the context of the emergency services – Issues in the use of counselling skills – Counselling skills in action – Working with post traumatic stress – Vicarious traumatization – Counselling skills in peer support – Legal and ethical implications in the use of counselling skills – Conclusion – Appendix A – Symptoms of Post Traumatic Stress Disorder – Appendix B – Secondary symptoms of Post Traumatic Stress Disorder – Appendix C – Symptoms of stress – Appendix D – Referral resources – References – Index.

129pp   0 335 20060 5 (Paperback)

COUNSELLING SKILLS FOR NURSES, MIDWIVES AND HEALTH VISITORS

Dawn Freshwater

This book is compact and easy to read, and could make a significant contribution to practitioners' ability to communicate effectively and make their practice patient centred.

Journal of Clinical Nursing

This is a delightful book which is well written, easy to read and suitable for students, qualified nurses and those who are specialist nurses.

Journal of Community Nursing

Counselling is a diverse activity and there are an increasing number of people who find themselves using counselling skills, not least those in the caring professions. There is a great deal of scope in using counselling skills to promote health in the everyday encounters that nurses have with their patients. The emphasis on care in the community and empowerment of patients through consumer involvement means that nurses are engaged in providing support and help to people to change behaviours.

This book examines contemporary developments in nursing and health care in relation to the fundamental philosophy of counselling, the practicalities of counselling and relevant theoretical underpinnings. Whilst the text is predominantly aimed at nurses, midwives and health visitors, it will also be of interest to those professionals allied to medicine, for example physiotherapists, occupational therapists and dieticians

Contents
Introduction – The process of counselling- Beginning a relationship – Sustaining the relationship – Facilitating change – Professional considerations – Caring for the carer – Appendix – Useful information – References – Index

122pp   0 335 20781 2 (paperback)

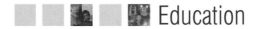
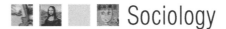
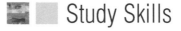
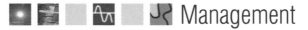
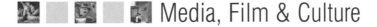
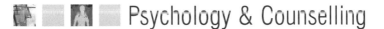
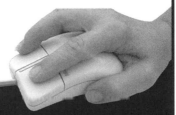